- Colds and flus start off with different symptoms, and recognizing them can help you choose the best remedy.

- A sneeze isn't the only way to spread a cold or the flu, so learn to spot the places the virus may be lurking. But the good news is . . . kissing doesn't spread the bug!

- Stress can double your chances of getting sick—especially right before an important event, but specific relaxation techniques can help you sail through the big day.

- Two delicious edible mushrooms may work magic with their antiviral effects.

- Aromatherapy can make a hot bath or a fragrant rub an effective cold and flu fighter.

- Vitamin C is a proven remedy . . . if you know how much to take and what mineral can boost its power.

FIND OUT MORE IN . . .
NATURAL MEDICINE FOR COLDS AND FLU

Books available from the Dell Natural Medicine Library:

NATURAL MEDICINE FOR HEART DISEASE

NATURAL MEDICINE FOR BREAST CANCER

NATURAL MEDICINE FOR ARTHRITIS

NATURAL MEDICINE FOR DIABETES

NATURAL MEDICINE FOR BACK PAIN

NATURAL MEDICINE FOR PROSTATE PROBLEMS

NATURAL MEDICINE FOR WEIGHT LOSS

NATURAL MEDICINE FOR COLDS AND FLU

NATURAL MEDICINE FOR PMS

NATURAL MEDICINE FOR SUPER IMMUNITY

THE DELL
NATURAL MEDICINE LIBRARY

NATURAL MEDICINE FOR
COLDS AND FLU

Nancy Pauline Bruning

Foreword by Timothy Kuss, Ph.D., C.N.C.

A Lynn Sonberg Book

A Dell Book

Published by
Dell Publishing
a division of
Bantam Doubleday Dell Publishing Group, Inc.
1540 Broadway
New York, New York 10036

IMPORTANT NOTE: Neither this nor any other book should be used as a substitute for professional medical care or treatment. It is advisable to seek the guidance of a physician or other qualified health practitioner before implementing any of the approaches to health suggested in this book. This book was written to provide selected information to the public concerning conventional and alternative medical treatments for colds and flu. Research in this field is ongoing and subject to interpretation. Although we have made all reasonable efforts to include the most up-to-date and accurate information in this book, there is no guarantee that what we know about this complex subject won't change with time. The reader should bear in mind that this book is not intended to take the place of medical advice from a trained medical professional. Readers are advised to consult a physician or other qualified health professional regarding treatment of all of their health problems. Neither the publisher, the producer, nor the author takes any responsibility for any possible consequences from any treatment, action, or application of medicine or preparation by any person reading or following the information in this book.

Table on pp. 64–72 from *The Real Vitamin & Mineral Book,* 2nd Ed. by Shari Lieberman and Nancy Bruning © 1997. Avery Publishing Group, Inc., Garden City Park, NY. Reprinted by permission.

Published by arrangement with
Lynn Sonberg Book Associates
10 West 86th Street
New York, NY 10024

Printed in the United States of America

Published simultaneously in Canada

June 1998

10 9 8 7 6 5 4 3 2 1

OPM

CONTENTS

FOREWORD

The average adult gets two to four colds per year; and each year 20,000 Americans die from complications due to flu. Much of this suffering is unnecessary and would vanish if more people used natural medicine. If you are among the growing number of individuals who wants above-average health and are interested in relieving cold and flu symptoms without side effects and boosting your resistance to these annoying infections, this is the book for you.

For the reader new to natural healing, *Natural Medicine for Colds and Flu* provides the basic introductory concepts of complementary medicine in simple, straightforward language. Ms. Bruning emphasizes a truly holistic approach to both the prevention and management of colds and flu by discussing the importance of food, vitamin and mineral supplements, herbs, homeopathy, and mind-body medicine. She provides you with the necessary tools and information to implement one or many of these strategies, and guides you toward safe, effective self-care as well as reputable professional care.

With each passing year, the demand for reliable information about natural medicine grows greater and greater. For example, month by month additional doctors and pharmacies join the ranks of those recommending natural medicine. And drugstores now routinely offer a wide selection of natural remedies such as herbs, vitamins, and homeopathics.

The growth of natural medicine has resulted from limits of conventional medicine. Nowhere is this better exemplified than in the treatment of colds and flu. As this book well documents, conventional medicine has been largely ineffective against many common ailments including these upper respiratory infections. Conventional medicine offers little in the way of prevention, and over-the-counter cold relief medications may do more harm than good. Most alarming of all, a recent survey found that half of patients with colds and other upper respiratory infections were given prescriptions for antibiotics. This translates into 12 million inappropriately issued prescriptions—antibiotics are worthless against the majority of these infections because they are caused by viruses, not bacteria. Antibiotics not only hamper the immune system; their misuse and overuse have created disease-resistant strains of bacteria—"supergerms"—that are more and more difficult to eliminate.

In contrast, natural medicines offer a host of benefits and are usually devoid of detrimental side effects. Natural medicines not only ease symptoms but can strengthen your resistance so you avoid infections in the future.

For example, the herb echinacea has made its reputation primarily via European research as an "immunostimulant." In 1992, two German studies determined that echinacea helped reduce the severity of colds and flu and helped people recover from them faster. In other studies, echinacea boosted T-lymphocyte activity and interferon, a natural substance vital to the body's defenses. In several dozen laboratory studies of viruses, including flu, herpes, and polio, a variety of active constituents of echinacea have demonstrated antiviral and immune-boosting activity. Combination herbal remedies that employ a variety of complementary and synergistic ingredients are even more effective, in my experience.

Another example is diet and nutrition. These twin approaches are of utmost importance in maintaining a vigilant immune response. Study after study has demonstrated an improvement in immune function in elderly people who take vitamin and mineral supplements, and vitamin C supplements have been shown to lessen symptoms and shorten the duration of a cold.

There are over 200 different types of cold and flu viruses in the air, on people's hands, and on everyday objects, waiting to gain entry into the human body. A living human body makes an ideal incubation chamber, providing all the essentials including food, shelter, and the right combination of temperature, water, and living cells that can be turned into virus replication factories.

But acting as the counterbalance is the immune response—the reason that when subjects are intentionally exposed to cold viruses, only one-half to two-thirds come down with colds, even though laboratory tests show they are all infected with the virus. The human body contains approximately 54 billion white blood cells whose mission is to destroy and devour viruses and other microbes. It is these white cells of the immune system that natural therapies enhance, providing protection and strength to resist and recover quickly.

As a complementary health professional myself, I applaud both the thoroughness of Ms. Bruning's research and her depth of understanding of the topic. You, the reader, will benefit greatly if you utilize the knowledge provided. *Natural Remedies for Cold and Flu* sets a new and higher standard for the relief and prevention of these common upper respiratory infections. Those of you who follow Ms. Bruning's advice will find yourselves healthier and most likely happier as you sidestep the aches and pains of the cold and flu. Furthermore, you will discover an extra week or two of health each year to be used in whatever way you desire! Just begin to imagine the possibilities. If you can imagine it, you have the ability to achieve it!

Timothy Kuss, Ph.D., C.N.C.
Pleasant Hill, California

INTRODUCTION

We usually think of the wintertime as the cold and flu season. But a cold can happen any time of the year, and in the United States the flu season extends from October through May. So perhaps you've begun to notice the first few warning signs—the scratchy throat, the headache, the sudden overwhelming sense of fatigue, that ache-all-over feeling. Perhaps people around you are dropping like flies, sniffling, sneezing, coughing, acting cranky. Or perhaps you feel fine now but want to start a prevention program. Either way, this book is for you.

The beauty of having a cold or flu is that you're never alone. Colds and flu are by far the most popular ailments ever to annoy the human race. Consider this:

- Colds are the number-one infectious illness worldwide.
- Colds account for more illness than all other diseases combined.
- The average adult gets two to four colds per year.
- Americans lose 30 million days of school and work each year because of colds.
- 7.9 million of our doctor visits are due to colds.
- We spend $1 billion on cold medicines each year.
- Five percent of Americans—12 million people—have a cold as you read this sentence.

- A flu can rip through a community in three weeks, affecting 20 to 50 percent of the population.
- Each year, 20,000 deaths are associated with the flu in the United States, due mostly to life-threatening complications.

We say "It's only a cold" or "a touch of the flu." And it's true that by themselves, these infections are not serious. But we should take them seriously because that's the only way to avoid them—and to avoid their leading to other serious infections, such as sinusitis, bronchitis, pneumonia, ear infections, or an attack of asthma. No wonder that throughout history, people have tried to beat these illnesses and come up with some rather weird remedies in the process, such as wearing necklaces of onions and garlic, dunking the feet in cold water, plastering the chest with mustard, wrapping the throat in salted herring, squirting sea water into the nose, and, of course, eating copious amounts of chicken soup.

These traditional folk remedies were the forerunners of today's natural medicines. Fortunately, we've come a long way since then. For example, whiskey is no longer the cold remedy of choice for Americans (although this custom persists to this day in the form of hot toddies and "nighttime" commercial remedies that contain surprising amounts of alcohol). Today many so-called traditional folk remedies—particularly herbs and other plant-based substances—are being validated by science and, thus, increasingly accepted by and available to the average person. More and more peer-reviewed medical journals are publishing articles and studies that support the use of natural medicines in strengthening the immune system in general and in easing symptoms of cold and flu in particular. No one knows for sure, but chances are that many more people are using natural therapies to manage symptoms of cold and flu than we might suspect.

We do know that in 1993, the *New England Journal of Medicine* published a survey that found that one out of three Americans used alternative care. We spent nearly $14 billion on complementary therapies, and 75 percent of that came out of our own pockets—not from our insurance companies. Today there are estimates that half of all Americans are using some form of alternative medicine and that we are spending $3 billion a year on vitamin supplements alone.

Books on natural or alternative medicine are best-sellers, including the book version of Bill Moyers's six-part public television series on mind-body healing. Natural medicines such as those featured in this book—diet and nutritional therapy, herbal therapy, homeopathy, acupuncture, relaxation therapies, massage—are gradually working their way into mainstream medicine. Courses in alternative medicine are being offered in some of the top medical schools in the country. We now have a federally funded Office of Alternative Medicine in Washington, and major medical institutions such as Columbia-Presbyterian Medical Center are offering hypnosis, guided imagery, yoga, and other alternative therapies along with conventional treatments.

Part of this surging popularity is a backlash against the deficiencies of conventional medicine. Although modern conventional medicine does have its success stories, we are growing increasingly frustrated and disenchanted with the way medicine is being practiced—and what it costs. Conventional medicine's main claim to fame—reduced deaths from epidemics and infectious diseases—in fact owes a great deal to improved sanitation, food storage and distribution, and living conditions. Even one of conventional medicine's most fabulous success stories—antibiotics to treat bacterial infection—is losing its luster. We have been overusing these "wonder drugs," which weakens their curative power by encouraging drug-resistant strains of bacteria to develop.

Instead of preventing disease effectively, or helping the body to heal the underlying disease, we take drugs that simply suppress disease symptoms. A perfect example is colds and flu. We treat something as mundane as the common cold by taking antibiotics, which are ineffective against viruses. We bombard it with cough suppressants and decongestants to get us through the first few days of the infection; then we spend the second half of the cold recuperating from the side effects of the drugs. Among the side effects of cold and flu medicines are drowsiness, dry mouth, headaches, elevated blood pressure, nausea, irregular heartbeat, blurred vision, skin rash, nervousness, and mood changes. Compare this with some of the "side effects" of natural therapies: lowered blood pressure, increased energy and stamina, greater mental clarity, reduced stress, improved digestion, and lowered risk of cancer and heart disease.

Where colds and flu are concerned, natural medicine is not just as good as conventional medicine; it is *better*. It is more effective and has more to offer. That's because natural medicine takes a totally different approach to healing. It is based on the concept that our bodies possess the innate wisdom to cure ourselves of disease and that the best medicine is one that works with the body's and the mind's natural processes. Unlike conventional medicine, natural medicine enhances your own natural immunity, and the best way to treat a cold or flu is to improve immune function. Unlike conventional medicine, it does not aim to suppress symptoms. This masking effect sometimes convinces us we are better but in reality does nothing to speed recovery; in fact, it actually may slow down the healing process.

For example, many people take aspirin to relieve muscle aches and fever during an illness. However, a Johns Hopkins University study compared people who took aspirin during a cold with those who did not. Symptoms in the aspirin-takers took a couple of days longer to clear up. While conventional medicine can slow recovery, natural medicine can speed it. In studies of the herb echinacea and studies of vitamin C supplements, those who took either one recovered faster than those who did not.

What This Book Can Do for You

Although vitamin C is the most popular natural cold remedy, and it has been shown to shorten a cold's duration, there's much more to natural cold and flu therapy than vitamin C. This book shows you the best way to use dozens of tried-and-true approaches including nutritional supplements, herbs, homeopathic remedies, and relaxation therapies. Learning about them and using them the right way may:

- Help you lessen the risk of getting a cold or flu
- Lessen the severity of symptoms if infection does take hold
- Shorten the duration of a cold or flu
- Prevent complications such as sinusitis, bronchitis, pneumonia, ear infection
- Help make sure your recovery is complete so symptoms don't linger and so you don't have a relapse

Thus this book is especially useful not just for those whose busy schedules would be interrupted by an upper respiratory infection but for people who must minimize risk of infection because they are at risk for complications due to colds and flu—the elderly, the chronically ill, moms-to-be, those with chronic lung disease including asthma, and those with other chronic diseases such as diabetes, heart disease, kidney disease, or cystic fibrosis.

From nutritional supplements to relaxation techniques, these therapies work. The first two chapters lay the groundwork for understanding and caring for a cold or flu. The book begins with an explanation of what colds and flus are, how they are spread, and how your immune system handles them. Is kissing okay? Why do kids get so many colds? Why does your nose run—or get congested? What are the possible complications of a cold or flu? Chapter 2 explains why conventional cold and flu medicines can cause more problems than they solve. Chapter 3 shows you how natural medicine can help your immune system function at its very best—here's where you'll find eight simple strategies for avoiding colds and flu. Chapter 4 gives you basic home care measures for taking care of yourself when you catch one of these bugs and eight no-nonsense strategies for beating a cold or flu.

The following chapters describe the most popular and effective natural therapies that are commonly available in the United States. Chapter 5 guides you in using everyday foods as medicine, from soups and herbal teas to immune-boosting mushrooms and garlic. The right foods in the right amounts can truly soothe and help heal. The next chapter, Chapter 6, explains why it's a good idea to augment your diet with nutritional supplements—whether you are sick and want to speed recovery, or whether you are well and want to improve your resistance. Chapter 7 covers herbal medicine and the amazing power of plants to heal and comfort. Chapter 8 covers homeopathy and helps you prescribe the correct remedy for each particular cold, flu, and person. The mind-body medicines in Chapter 9 will help you enlist your innate healer using the latest ways to manage stress and make that all-important connection between our inner and outer self.

Once you have become acquainted with this basic information, you'll be ready to turn to Chapter 10, "Putting It All Together"; this chapter succinctly outlines specific programs using all the natural therapies to stop a cold or flu at the first sign, to shorten the duration and lessen symptoms in the middle of one, and to lessen your chances of getting sick in the first place.

Experiment to see which approaches best fit your life view and lifestyle, and which is most effective. If you are pleased with the results, perhaps you'll be encouraged to use natural therapies to prevent and treat other illnesses.

Whether you use natural therapies on your own or under the guidance of a health professional, an open discussion with your conventional doctor can benefit you both. The 1993 survey mentioned on page xv showed not only that one-third of Americans used alternative care, it indicated that they were reluctant to share this information with their doctors. This finding took many conventional physicians by surprise and thus was a long-overdue wake-up call. Today you are less likely to be rebuffed, or ignored, or patronized when talking about "alternatives" such as herbs and vitamin supplements. You owe it to your doctor to inform him or her about your other health practices and interests; and he or she owes it to you to listen with an open mind. Show your doctor this book and point out the evidence that natural therapies work.

A Word to the Wise

Dozens of natural therapies from a host of different cultures have helped people around the world manage cold and flu symptoms. Many of the natural remedies are based on centuries of use and observation, and we're learning more about these therapies as more studies are being done. These therapies are generally quite safe. But remember: Just because a remedy is considered to be "natural" doesn't mean it is *guaranteed* to be safe. Some remedies are quite powerful, and some have serious side effects if taken inappropriately or in toxic amounts. The remedies in this book have been found to be safe for most people when taken in the recommended amounts. However, the safest course of action is to consult your health care provider before trying any natural therapy, especially if you are under the care of a physician for a diagnosed medical condition. Also remember that if you try a natural remedy and your condition becomes worse, or if you notice any unwanted effects, discontinue the treatment and seek professional help, either from your conventional doctor or from a qualified natural health specialist.

CHAPTER ONE

Understanding Colds and Flu

Both colds and flu are minor infections of the respiratory system that occur when viruses invade your cells and multiply. (See Figure 1.1.) To be sure, they are annoying and sometimes debilitating. They even can lead to other, more serious infections. But many natural medicine practitioners feel that a cold or flu actually can be a positive thing. They reason that these minor infections are nature's way of warning you that your body is too weak to throw off cold and flu viruses, and this could be a sign that your body is heading toward other more serious diseases.

If you succumb every year to one or more "bugs," it could mean it's time to slow down, eat better, and make other health-building changes in your life. In that sense, colds and flu are not the enemy; they are your allies. By preventing colds and flu and strengthening your response to them, you are doing yourself another favor as well—increasing your all-around health.

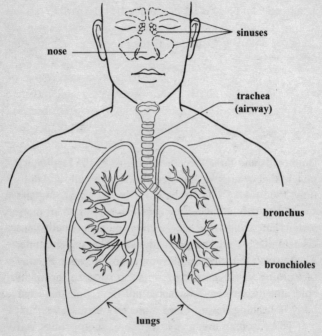

Figure 1.1

Is It a Cold or Flu?

Although it doesn't really matter for overall treatment purposes, if you're like most people, you want to know whether you've got a cold or the flu. Oftentimes a cold is brushed off as "just" a cold, but the flu is more serious and elicits more sympathy. Sometimes it's hard to tell one from the other, but in most cases, the following guide should help you make the distinction.

- It's likely you have a *cold* if the symptoms come on slowly and affect primarily the head and throat: a mild to moderate cough, sneezing, a stuffy nose, and swollen sinuses. Any fatigue or achy feeling is generally mild. There's usually no headache unless your sinuses are involved, and no fever or only a low fever in adults.
- You know you have the *flu* if the infection arrives suddenly, affects the bronchial tubes and lungs, and causes you to feel awful all over. A flu usually causes a cough that may be severe and very painful and exhaustion that may come on suddenly and last for two weeks. You may have an all-over achy feeling that may be severe, headache, and fever that may reach 102 degrees F or more and last for up to four days. Only occasionally does a flu cause sneezing, stuffy nose, or congested sinuses.
- Although some people experience nausea, vomiting, or diarrhea during a flu, these symptoms are rarely prominent. The term "stomach flu" sometimes is incorrectly used to describe gastrointestinal illnesses caused by other microorganisms, food poisoning, excess alcohol, or other causes, and which usually goes away in a day or two.

Is It Viral or Bacterial?

Another source of confusion about upper respiratory infections is whether they are viral or bacterial in nature. In natural medicine, again, the distinction is not that important because viral infections such as colds and flu and bacterial infections are generally all treated the same way. That's because the goal is mainly to boost immune function so your body can heal itself and destroy the invaders. However, treatment sometimes can be tailored more specifically. For example, some herbs also seek to affect the virus directly, and certain other herbs are better known for their antibacterial properties. Generally:

- If the mucus is clear or white, the infection is probably viral in nature; head colds are due to viral infections, as are flus.
- If you have green mucus and symptoms are localized to the throat, lungs, or sinuses, your infection is probably bacterial in nature; bronchitis and sinusitis often fall into this category.

Sometimes you can have both viral and bacterial infections simultaneously, and one also can lead to the other. Often a cold or flu is confused with sinusitis, and sometimes a viral infection can lead to a bacterial infection of the sinuses and vice versa. If you seek medical help, your practitioner will aim to diagnose your condition more precisely in order to choose a treatment with specific antiviral or antibacterial action. The distinction is more important in conventional medicine because bacterial infections usually are treated with antibiotics, which are not effective against viruses. (More about this later.)

Symptoms—Annoying but Necessary

Viruses themselves do not produce any symptoms. Rather, coughs, runny noses, aches, and fevers are signs that your immune system is responding to an overgrowth of viruses. It is ironic that we don't realize that we've "caught" a cold or flu until days after the virus has been transmitted, when our bodies have begun to deal with it.

That's why in natural medicine, symptoms are never confused with the disease itself. Instead, think of them as your body's best efforts to deal with a disease—your body's unique way of expressing that a disease is present and that it is mounting a defense against the disease.

An oft-cited example of our healing ability is the use of fever. When bacteria or viruses grow out of control, your body responds by creating fever. The higher temperature accomplishes several things: It spurs the production of an antiviral substance called interferon; it increases the activity of your white blood cells, which fight infections; and it slows down the activity of bacteria, making them more susceptible to attack. Natural medicine has long appreciated fever as a powerful natural healing mechanism that your ailing body "knows" to produce.

Conventional medicine is only beginning to realize that unless your fever is raging so high that it could cause harm, a high temperature should not be lowered artificially with drugs such as aspirin or acetaminophen. Doing so actually could prolong the course of the infection (and giving aspirin to children could lead to a dangerous condition called Reye's syndrome). Other examples include coughing, which helps clear breathing tubes and rid the body of mucus and dead pathogens; diarrhea, which speeds the evacuation of pathogens and irritants from the bowel; and vomiting, which empties the stomach of harmful or poisonous substances.

So, although they may make you feel uncomfortable or worse, symptoms are really a sign that your body is doing its job to restore your health. Clobbering a cold with conventional drugstore or prescription medicines, which suppresses symptoms, actually can thwart the body's natural ability to fight off the bug. Natural remedies gently soothe symptoms by working with—not against—your body's natural processes while encouraging the body to heal itself.

How You "Catch" a Cold or Flu

Cold and flu viruses survive and spread because humans are a social species, and one that likes to travel. Scientists think that cold viruses first appeared when humans were still hunter-gatherers, living in small groups that rarely mingled. At that point in history, cold viruses fought hard to survive, spread, and multiply, as demonstrated by modern-day experience with scientists who live in a research station in Antarctica. These isolated souls have no contact with outsiders once the summer visitors leave. Those remaining catch the one or two colds left behind, and, in time, everyone becomes immune to those particular viruses. The viruses die out, and colds simply don't happen. That is, until the next spring, when visitors inadvertently deposit new viruses. In order to survive and spread, cold viruses apparently need fairly large numbers of people and travelers that carry the virus from place to place.

Because of our modern civilization and the survival mechanisms developed by the virus, today people are walking, talking, sneezing, coughing, touching agents of contamination. They may be shedding viruses as soon as within seven hours of initial infection; however, transmission usually peaks as symptoms begin or are at their height, and may continue for a week to ten days after symptoms have subsided—and for up to four weeks in children. Often a person may develop a low-grade infection with symptoms that are so mild as to be unnoticeable, yet still the virus may be shed and spread to others—in other words, you can be exposed to viruses by people who are not sick themselves.

How do cold and flu viruses get from one person to another? Beginning with Louis Pasteur's discovery of infectious microorganisms, scientists suspected these viruses were spread when people sneezed or coughed. We now know that each of these little explosions propels droplets containing millions of viruses into the air, which the unsuspecting healthy person inhales.

The airborne mode of transmission was proven once and for all by Elliot Dick, Ph.D., a cold researcher at the University of Wisconsin, who began staging experiments involving poker games in the 1980s. In one early experiment, he sequestered healthy college students into a suite of rooms and then added a few people with colds. They then played poker for one week in these close quarters. Not surprisingly, all the healthy students caught colds—along with about half the researchers. However, in another experiment, only 20 percent of the healthy subjects became infected, leading Dr. Dick to conclude that the virus is spread by the air but that it wasn't necessarily that easy to catch.

Flu viruses, on the other hand, are easier to catch. For example, after a mere three-hour airplane flight, a person who had the flu had infected almost three-fourths of the other passengers. Many people report that they get upper respiratory infections after flying, and airlines have admitted that as an economy measure, they have reduced the inflow of fresh air into planes during flights, so stale air that may have a high concentration of viruses is being recirculated.

Other researchers have found another means of upper respiratory virus transmission. Jack Gwaltney, M.D., of the University of Virginia in Charlottesville, found that infected people pick up live viruses on their hands when they touch their noses. If they then touch such common nonporous objects as doorknobs, telephones, and money, they transfer the virus to those objects. There the virus lies in wait for other people to pick up on their hands when they touch the same objects; those people then infect themselves when they touch their noses or eyes. (If a virus enters the tear duct in the corner of your eye, it can reach the back of your throat via a small connecting tube.)

WHAT ABOUT KISSING?

Kissing, you'll be thankful to know, doesn't transmit the cold virus. Dr. Elliot Dick's work at Respiratory Virus Research Laboratory proved that as well. Thirteen pairs of volunteers, one of each pair infected with a particular cold virus, smooched for a minute to a minute and a half. Just one healthy subject caught a cold. Dr. Jack Gwaltney, however, points out that—outside the laboratory, at least—kissers are usually touchers too. So if one partner's hand picks up a virus from the other and then touches his or her own nose or eyes, a cold or flu might ensue.

Knowing how these viruses are transmitted can help you avoid being exposed to cold and flu viruses and, it is hoped, cut down on your risk of becoming infected. In the following chapter, you'll find specific steps to take to avoid coming into contact with these pesky pathogens in the first place.

What Are Viruses?

Viruses are not at all like bacteria. Although they often are referred to as tiny organisms, these particles are not really alive. They are mere fragments of genetic material known as RNA (ribonucleic acid) or DNA (deoxyribonucleic acid) surrounded by a shell of protein. Viruses do not eat, breathe, grow, or repair themselves. They can live and reproduce only in living cells. A single virus is about 1/100th the size of a bacterium; imagine something so tiny that about 10,000 of them can fit on the head of a pin!

Viruses are programmed to invade only specific cells in specific animals (called *hosts*), such as humans. They gain entry because they have little "keys" on their surfaces that fit into "locks" on the cell surface. Once a viral key enters a lock, called a *receptor,* the cell opens up and bingo! like a safe cracker, the virus is in. The virus then springs into life, taking over the cell and forcing it to reproduce thousands of new viruses, which then go on to invade more cells and produce more copies of themselves, spreading the infection. Unlike bacteria, viruses hide inside cells, so killing them with drugs is difficult and risks injuring or killing the cells.

Types of Cold and Flu Viruses

Colds and flu are caused by over 200 different kinds of viruses. That's why it's been impossible to create a vaccine to prevent these infections—vaccines work only against a single organism or a group of organisms that are closely related. Seven major families of viruses cause upper respiratory infection. The three main families are rhinoviruses, parainfluenza viruses, and corona viruses.

One family, the corona family, causes flu, and the remaining six families cause the common cold. Each cold or flu virus is capable of causing a slightly different cold or flu, with slightly different symptoms. We usually associate colds and flu with wintertime, but as a group, these viruses are active all year round, and many viruses are active at the same time of year. Over the course of a nine-month study, researchers found 14 different rhinoviruses in a single Chicago nursery school.

Your Immune Defense System at Work

So, what happens once a virus lands on your unsuspecting body?

When healthy, your body has a formidable defense system, including the membranes that line the respiratory passageways as well as the immune system. The immune system is composed of the lymphatic system, which includes the thymus gland, spleen, tonsils, and lymph nodes and vessels. In addition, you have specialized cells that pump out chemicals, send signals to other immune cells and the brain, tag infected cells, kill viruses and cells, and eat the tattered remains.

Unwelcome pathogens first encounter simple cellular mechanisms designed to keep our bodies as "germ-free" as possible. Let's look at the nose, the prime entry point, since you inhale and exhale about 23,000 times a day, often through your nose. Nature, in its wisdom, has made the environment inside your nose quite inhospitable to viruses. In the first place, its ample blood supply close to the surface warms the incoming air to approximate body temperature as it moistens it. Viruses don't like warm, moist air—they prefer it dry and cool.

Second, your nose and throat also are lined with a mucous membrane (called mucosa) whose job it is to secrete a protective layer of mucus—between one pint and one quart per day. As you inhale, particles such as viruses, bacteria, pollen, and dust stick to the mucus and become trapped. These cells also have tiny hairs called *cilia,* which are designed to sweep mucus and foreign particles toward the back of your nose and windpipe and down your food pipe. (See Figure 1.2.) When these particles reach your stomach, digestive acids destroy most of the potential troublemakers. If the virus comes into contact with your eye, tear ducts may be able to wash away organisms or pass them on to the cilia and mucosa to deal with.

Cells along your respiratory tract also secrete *antibodies.* These specialized proteins latch onto the viruses, altering the shape of their "keys" so they no longer fit the "locks" of the target cells. The specific type of antibody that prevents cold and flu viruses from taking hold is called *immunoglobulin A (IgA),* but, as any cold sufferer knows, viruses occasionally penetrate this first line of defense.

When this happens, the target cells in the upper respiratory tract allow the virus to inject its genetic material, turning the cell into a hapless virus factory. Each infected cells is capable of churning out thousands of copies of the invading virus, infecting the nose and throat. The infection triggers the cells to release messenger chemicals that in turn set into motion an amazing chain of immunological events.

The initial chemicals, called *prostaglandins,* cause in-

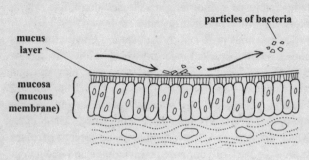

Figure 1.2

flammation in the infected area, so within the first week after the virus has penetrated a cell, you feel the first symptom—a sore scratchy throat, perhaps a slight headache, and the vague feeling that you're coming down with something. Prostaglandins also summon forth the white blood cells called *neutrophils.* These specialized cells try to engulf the replicating viruses and digest them. As the neutrophils do their work, the infected area becomes more inflamed. The blood vessels dilate, and more blood plasma floods the area, bringing more white cells as well as additional warmth, which slows down the virus replication.

Meanwhile, your body also releases *histamine.* This chemical boosts production of mucus to trap more viruses and enhance the flooding of plasma and white cells to the area. Some of the plasma leaks into the mucous membranes lining the nose and throat, causing more swelling. As a result, you get that stuffed-up feeling. Not only is it uncomfortable for you to breathe, but the extra mucus brought on by the histamine can't take its usual route down the throat and into your digestive system for disposal. With nowhere else to go, the mucus runs out of your nose, and thus begins the endless stream of tissues and nose-blowing. Nerves in your nose sense the swelling, and the brain signals your body to sneeze. Nerves in your throat also sense the extra mucus and force you to cough, expelling the mucus before it can get to the lungs. Your throat gets sore from the inflammation, coughing, and mouth breathing due to your stuffy nose. Your lymph nodes may swell—a sign that they are producing more cells and trapping the virus.

This first stage of response generally lasts four to five hours. Should it fail to beat the virus, your body switches into the next gear. Other white blood cells are called to the scene. One type, the *monocytes,* become *macrophages,* which help the neutrophils gobble up the viruses. Macrophages are also responsible for releasing *interleukin-1,* a chemical that raises your body temperature, causing fever. Often the body lags behind the brain's signal to give the virus the heat treatment. The discrepancy between wish and reality causes the "chills" you sometimes get before a fever. Interleukin-1 is also the body chemical that causes that achy feeling, which is due to the breakdown of protein in your muscles.

Finally, interleukin-1 summons another type of white blood cell, the *lymphocytes.* As they emerge from their home bases in the lymph glands, lymphocytes are transformed. One type of lymphocyte, the *B-cells* (so named because they mature your bone marrow), produces immunoglobulins. Remember, IgA blocks viruses from the cells' receptor sites. Some of the B-cells turn into "memory cells"—they "remember" the virus and are able to recognize it the next time your body encounters it. Another lymphocyte, the *T-cells,* matures in the thymus gland. Some of them are transformed into killer cells that destroy cells that have been infected with the virus, effectively shutting down the factory. Some turn into helper cells that encourage B-cells to churn out more antibodies. And some eventually become suppressor cells whose sole purpose is to turn on the immune response once the coast is clear.

The incubation period—the time between being exposed to a virus and the onset of symptoms due to infection—varies from one to six days. The battle itself—during which the virus and its clones are destroyed—lasts a week or ten days. Since the immune cells are no longer needed by the body, your symptoms subside as those cells return to their home bases, ready to do battle with the next pesky invader.

Who Gets Sick and Why?

Why is it that some people get every little cold and flu that comes along, while other people never or almost never succumb?

According to natural medicine, infections such as colds and flu are nothing more than parasites living off the human organism. Many of these parasites or ''germs'' are ubiquitous in our lives and in our bodies and normally do not cause problems until for some reason they grow out of control. Others are rare or new to our lives and catch us by surprise.

More than ''Germs''

Natural medicine believes that the ''germ theory'' plays a role in determining who will succumb to infection and how severe it will be. This theory includes the notion that the frequency and volume of exposure matter: Everyone is at higher risk during an epidemic or the flu season, or in a situation such as a day care center where germs are plentiful and passed easily by close and frequent contact. Another factor is the relative invasiveness and infectiveness of the parasite: Some critters simply are stronger and more aggressive than others, and an organism such as a virus tends to gain strength during the course of an invasion.

But obviously it is not simply a matter of being exposed to a virus or other *pathogen* (an organism or substance that produces disease). This was obvious even to Louis Pasteur, the father of the "germ theory" of disease. On his deathbed, he is reported to have said "The germ is nothing—the terrain is everything." What he meant is that germs alone do not cause disease because they cannot invade a healthy body, or "terrain." We are not helpless victims just waiting to be colonized by very little aliens. Most of the time, people can resist infection. In order for a pathogen to take hold and colonize, you must have some chink in your armor—your immune system must be deficient or overly stressed in some way.

Natural medicine therefore also gives great weight to the susceptibility of the "host" to its "guests." Your infection is not caused solely by the presence of a parasite; rather, it is the result of a previously established disease that leaves you more susceptible. Susceptibility explains why some people rarely get colds, flu, or other infectious diseases, even while nursing the sick, and why others "catch everything" and suffer multiple colds during the year.

Everything in nature has a purpose, although that purpose may not always be clear to us. If you get a lot of colds or flus or take forever to recuperate from them, that is nature's signal that something is amiss with the ecology of your terrain. Many factors account for the tremendous variety in susceptibility to colds and flu, including psychological and physical stress, nutrition, and heredity. Interestingly, women contract more colds than men throughout their lives. It is theorized that this is due, at least in part, to the fact that women tend to be around children more than men (see below). Women also tend to be more susceptible to colds around the time of ovulation, probably because hormone fluctuations affect immunity.

As you'll see in subsequent chapters, natural medicine offers many ways to change your terrain and set your body right again. Through general lifestyle practices, improving your diet and nutrition, using healing herbs and homeopathic remedies, and reducing stress with mind-body therapies your body will better resist infection in the first place and recover more quickly should an infection take hold.

Kids and Colds

Children catch more colds than adults. Typical infants suffer as many as nine colds from birth to their first birthday. By the time they reach the age of three, they get about six per year. For one thing, young children's immune systems are less developed, and they simply don't have the equipment to fight infection. Second, they haven't been on the planet long enough to acquire the immunity to specific colds and flu viruses that adults have. Then, too: How many kids have you met who wash their hands and keep their fingers away from their noses? Yet those are two key measures to reduce exposure to viruses. Since kids are such potent breeding grounds for viruses, adults who spend a lot of time around children tend to catch more viruses too. But in time, adults become immune and the number of colds and flus they catch drops down. And children in day care, who, according to one study, get 60 percent more colds than kids who stay home, also eventually come out ahead. As time passed, and the toddlers in the study got older, they actually suffered half as many colds as the stay-at-home children.

The maturing process continues to work in your favor. During adolescence, the number of annual colds drops down to three or four. The risk continues to fall, until by the time you are a healthy elderly person, you get only about one or two colds a year, and they tend to be less severe.

Complications

Colds and flus certainly create discomfort and lost days from school and work and pleasure. But they are generally benign infections—minor disturbances that usually go away on their own and leave no permanent ill effects. However, they can lead to secondary infections in those with compromised immune systems or chronic respiratory problems. For example, these days it is common for children to develop ear infections as a result of a cold, for many people with weak sinuses to develop sinusitis, and for those with weak lungs to develop bronchitis. Flu epidemics in the past have killed many people, and it is still common for elderly people to contract pneumonia after a flu. According to the Centers for Disease Control and Prevention, in an average season, flu is associated with 20,000 deaths in this country; most of these deaths are among the elderly.

How can you avoid these dangerous complications? Drugs are not the answer, for most people. There are no effective antiviral medications suitable for colds and flu. Current conventional cold and flu medications only give symptom relief, and it is unwise to give antibiotics as a preventive measure. (See the next chapter.) The best course is to take care of yourself and use natural therapies to bolster your immune system so minor viral infections stay minor and go away quickly. With the appropriate natural care, a cold or flu can leave your immune system in better shape and you are less likely to suffer complications. And if you do suffer complications, there are natural remedies that can be used alone or in conjunction with conventional medicines to give all-round better care.

CHAPTER TWO

The Problem with Conventional Medicine

So, you've got a miserable cold or flu. You're sneezing, sniffling, aching, coughing . . . and you simply *must* finish that final report at work, or your youngest daughter is getting married. If you're tempted to take conventional medicine to get rid of your symptoms, think twice. Most of the mainstream remedies don't work very well, and many people who take them don't find any relief at all. And consider this: You not only run the risk of side effects but of prolonging your infection. You may be worse off than if you took nothing, particularly if you opt for one of those fancy combination remedies or if you take an antibiotic, which is only effective against bacteria, not viruses.

Not Worth the Price

You pay twice when you use a conventional cold or flu medicine.

You pay with your money. Over-the-counter cold medications are a $4 billion annual business worldwide, with

Americans spending half that amount. There are over 2,800 over-the-counter (OTC) products from which to choose. This array is so overwhelming that, while a person typically takes 53 seconds to choose the average OTC medicine, he or she needs a whopping two and a half minutes to pick out a cold medication, according to a market research firm. As the consumer, you need to realize that eye-grabbing labels and bogus distinctions disguise the fact that only a few ingredients actually work, and not very well at that. Natural remedies are generally much less expensive—and they are more effective.

You also pay with your health: Conventional medicines ''work'' by suppressing the symptoms without treating the underlying disease that produces the symptoms. Such suppression is like smashing a beeping smoke alarm instead of putting out the fire. The smoke alarm is a sign that something is wrong and needs to be attended to. Attending to the superficial warning fixes the immediate problem of annoying beeps but will not repair the underlying problem, which will only lead to greater problems later on.

Natural medicine practitioners have long argued against symptom suppression because minor infection may be an acute, self-limiting disease that is part of normal living and serves actually to strengthen the immune system. Natural remedies ease symptoms gently yet effectively and support your body's natural ability to fight infections; conventional drugs do not. Two Canadian researchers reviewed dozens of studies of OTC cold remedies and found that they neither attack cold viruses nor boost immunity— and therefore do not shorten the duration of a cold. A recent study supports this view—at least in the case of several nonprescription pain- and fever-reducing medications. The study showed that compared with people who took a placebo (dummy pill), people who took the medications experienced suppressed immune system response to the virus, a longer duration of infection, and more respiratory discomfort. So your health could suffer in both the short term and long term if you take these medicines. As you'll see in later chapters, natural remedies—such as vitamin C supplements and the herb echinacea—have been proven in studies to shorten the duration of colds and flu and have other health benefits as well.

The Trouble with . . .

Taking a single-action cold remedy can cause trouble because of unwanted side effects.

- *Decongestants:* Decongestants constrict your blood vessels, which reduces swelling and opens nasal passages. Decongestants taken in pill form stimulate the central nervous system, so you might get side effects of jumpiness and insomnia. Some also may raise your blood pressure significantly; people with high blood pressure should avoid them. Nasal sprays are more effective than pills, have fewer or no systemic side effects, and work fast. But if used longer than three days they may cause dependence and the rebound effect, where you end up feeling more stuffed up than before, and the drug no longer works.
- *Antihistamines:* Cold products that claim to dry up a runny nose usually contain an antihistamine, which is effective for allergies but is ineffective for most colds. Side effects may include dry eyes, nose, and mouth; impaired motor skills; and drowsiness that prevents you from driving or operating machinery.
- *Antitussives:* These cough suppressants suppress the

cough center of your brain. They may cause dizziness, drowsiness, nausea, and constipation.

- *Expectorants:* These are supposed to loosen phlegm and help you cough it up. Side effects may include nausea, headache, drowsiness, and confusion.

Combination Remedies: A Must to Avoid

Most of all, avoid those fancy combination remedies. In the first place, symptoms don't hit you all at once. Usually the first sign is a scratchy sore throat, perhaps some achiness. Then you feel congested, then your nose starts to run, and then you begin to cough and sneeze. Second, they often contain ingredients that are known to be ineffective for cold or flu. For example, they may contain an antihistamine, which won't help your runny nose but will make you drowsy. Third, they may contain surprising ingredients that you don't want to take, so read the label carefully. A common ingredient in liquid formulas is alcohol—some are 80 proof, as intoxicating as a shot of scotch. The commonly used decongestant phenylpropanolamine can raise blood pressure. Why subject your body to chemicals it doesn't need and that might cause unpleasant side effects? Why get locked into taking fixed amounts of the various ingredients, when you need the flexibility to vary the dosage as your symptoms wax and wane? And why take a product that may contain dueling ingredients, as is the case with Vicks 44E syrup, which contains an ingredient that loosens phlegm to make it easier to cough up and another one that's a cough suppressant?

What About Antibiotics?

For most people, there's no reason to get a doctor's prescription for antibiotics since they are useful only against bacteria, and colds and flu are caused by viruses. And there are plenty of reasons to avoid antibiotics.

Overuse and misuse of antibiotics have caused resistant strains of bacteria to develop, rendering these drugs useless for future use. Bacteria become resistant because of mutations that arise spontaneously. During antibiotic therapy, the nonresistant bacteria die off, leaving the resistant bacteria to flourish. Resistant bacteria then can transfer their antibiotic-resistant genetic material to other strains of bacteria, so they become resistant too. In a single day, one of these supergerms can reproduce 16 billion more of its bad self. That's why doctors may have to try several different antibiotics until they find one that is still effective against a particular bacterium; however, some strains of bacteria are completely resistant to *all* antibiotics currently available. The number of these resistant bacteria is growing so fast that this phenomenon has been dubbed "the coming plague." You may be astonished to learn that half of the antibiotics used in the United States are given to food animals and 90 percent of those are given for disease prevention and to promote growth. Many experts believe that this practice may be contributing to the wave of antibiotic-resistant bacteria. According to the Centers for Disease Control and Prevention, each year 19,000 hospital patients die of bacterial infections that are resistant to all available antibiotics.

Surveys have shown that antibiotics are being misused by both doctors and patients. In 1996 the American Lung Association commissioned a Gallup survey of 1,010 adults and 100 physicians. The physicians said that 70 percent of their patients inappropriately ask for antibiotics when they have a cold or flu. In the same survey, 60 percent of patients thought antibiotics were effective against viruses, and many believed that it was a good idea to take antibiotics during a cold or flu to prevent complications such as sinusitis, ear infection, or bronchitis. In another survey of Boston pediatricians, 71 percent said that at least four times in the last month a parent had asked them for an antibiotic unnecessarily; 35 percent said they sometimes comply, even though they know they shouldn't.

Yet research shows that when a healthy person takes antibiotics, it can change the distribution and resistance patterns of microorganisms already present in the body. Antibiotics prescribed to eradicate a certain bacterium can also kill friendly bacteria, such as those required to digest food and produce certain vitamins. Other bacteria, normally held in check, may thrive, setting you up for an infection in the future that the antibiotic won't cure. Furthermore, antibiotics often have troublesome side effects, including nausea and diarrhea, and some people are highly allergic to the drugs.

That's why antibiotics should be considered only for special cases, when you develop a bacterial infection such as sinusitis, an ear infection, or strep throat that has been confirmed by a throat culture. (Acute bronchitis, which is usually a viral infection, should not be treated with antibiotics.)

Even when a bacterial infection is present, the decision is not always clear-cut. Most of the antibiotics prescribed outside of hospitals in the U.S. are for childhood ear infection. But a study published in the May 24, 1997, issue of the *British Medical Journal* concluded that antibiotics provide only a "modest benefit" to children with ear infection. The authors analyzed six placebo-controlled clinical trials and found that antibiotics did not relieve pain during the first 24 hours any better than the placebo (dummy pill). A small group (14 percent) of untreated children still had pain two to seven days after being seen by the doctor; if these children received antibiotics, about 40 percent of them would have had less pain. What this means is that for every 17 children who get treated early with antibiotics, one would be prevented from having pain for two to seven days, and 16 children would undergo antibiotic treatment unnecessarily, since their pain would go away without treatment. In exchange, all 17 children undergo the risk of side effects such as diarrhea, vomiting, and rashes. The authors also found that antibiotics did not reduce the incidence of subsequent ear infections or deafness. Some experts believe that overuse of antibiotics in children three years or younger actually will impair their immunity. In fact, studies do demonstrate that antibiotics may lead to chronic ear infections. Since ear infections go away without any antibiotic treatment at all, some countries have made an effort to reduce excessive use of antibiotics. In the Netherlands, for example, only 31 percent of doctors prescribe antibiotics to children with ear infections, and children there have a remarkably low rate of antibiotic-resistant infections.

However, antibiotics do have a place in a small number of people with colds or flu. Antibiotics should be considered for preventive use in people who are prone to recurrent bacterial infection because their airways have been damaged by lung or bronchial disease and in people who are immune-deficient and are exposed to certain bacterial diseases.

* * *

If you do take an antibiotic, keep the following in mind:

- Be sure to take the entire course of pills. In the Gallup survey, more than half the patients did not finish the course, and most of them said they stopped because they were concerned they would develop resistance to the drug. Yet the opposite is true: Failure to take enough antibiotic, along with inappropriate use of antibiotics, is what makes the bacteria resistant.
- During the course of antibiotics, replenish and nourish the "good bacteria" by taking acidophilus, bifidus, and other beneficial bacteria, available in liquid and capsule form at health food stores. Fermented foods such as yogurt and miso also may restore beneficial bacteria.

CHAPTER THREE

Preventing Colds and Flu

The average person gets two to four colds a year—but who says you have to be average? Getting sick every year isn't inevitable—if you make a few adjustments in your daily habits. This chapter gives you eight easy ways to boost your resistance and be a "bad host" to cold and flu germs, from paying attention to the food you eat to the amount of exercise, rest, and sleep you get. You'll also find guidelines that will help you decide whether a flu vaccination is the right thing for you. In the following chapters, you'll find specific natural therapies that will boost immunity further, but your daily life activities are the foundation of a cold-and-flu-prevention program and the best place to start.

Eight Strategies to Boost Immunity

Follow these basic guidelines and you'll lower your risk of colds and flu and other infectious diseases as well as lessen the severity and duration of your symptoms if you do get sick. These basic steps also will improve your all-round health and make you fitter, stronger, and more energetic.

Strategy #1: Watch Out for Stress

It's quite common for someone to get a cold or flu at the worst possible time: while studying for a big exam, while under a crushing deadline, before a big presentation. This is not just coincidence or an active imagination. In a study at Carnegie-Mellon University, 400 subjects had live cold viruses put directly up their noses. Those who were under the highest amounts of stress, according to psychological testing, had double the rate of infection than those with the lowest stress.

It's been discovered that it's not just the big events that hamper your ability to resist a cold or flu. Even little daily hassles such as getting stuck in traffic can take their toll on your immune system; on the other hand, little "ups" such as compliments from others or friendly hugs can help you fend off colds.

So watch your stress levels, do your best to avoid situations that you *know* press your stress buttons, and try to increase the little pleasures in your day. And consider using some of the specific techniques in Chapter 9 to relax and better manage the stress in your life.

Strategy #2: Get Enough Rest

There is ample evidence that we are running up a huge "sleep debt" in this country. The average person needs between eight and nine hours of quality sleep—that is, uninterrupted sleep that goes through the normal cycles of heavy to light. During the deeper stages, your body repairs itself; during the light phases in which dreaming occurs, you release stress and tension.

If you need an alarm clock to get you up in the morning, you are not getting enough sleep. Without the rest that sleep affords, your body can't recover from daily stresses and your immune system suffers. Lack of sleep doesn't just make you cranky, forgetful, unproductive, and slow to react while driving or operating machinery. According to surveys, insomniacs get sick more frequently and take longer to recuperate.

If you have trouble getting enough sleep, reevaluate your priorities and investigate "sleep hygiene"—measures to help you get to sleep and stay asleep. These include: reducing your caffeine intake, especially late in the day; avoiding heavy meals at night; scheduling a quiet "wind-down" time before bedtime; using earplugs; making the room as dark as possible; going to sleep and getting up at the same time every day; and reserving your bed for sleeping and sex—not reading, watching TV, or working. In addition, there are several natural remedies to help you fall asleep and sleep soundly, including herbs and homeopathic remedies; the relaxation techniques in Chapter 9 also have helped many people.

Strategy #3: Be Physically Active

Many studies show that moderate exercise keeps your immune system humming and vigilant. For example, in a study of sedentary women, the group that added a brisk 45-minute walk to their daily routine experienced improved immune function and cut the number of days with cold symptoms in half. A follow-up study with a similar exercise pattern found that 50 percent of the nonexercisers caught colds but only 21 percent of the walkers came down with the bug during the study. And only 8 percent of the women who had been exercising before the study began caught colds.

Moderate exercise seems to optimize resistance by increasing the circulating white blood cells temporarily, but long enough to keep invaders under control. It also seems to stave off the immune system decline that goes hand in hand with aging; 65-year-olds in the second study had the T-cell count of 30-year-olds. But don't overdo it. Other studies show that a too-strenuous exercise program actually can depress the immune system. Elite athletes such as marathon runners are notoriously prone to colds and flu. Walking is the easiest, simplest, and best way to kick off a more active life; it's also a terrific mainstay no matter what else you do. Let your body be your guide and begin slowly, gradually increasing the distance and/or the intensity with which you cover the same distance. A good goal is brisk walking for two or three miles every other day; every day is preferable. Whatever you choose, make sure you enjoy it or can learn to enjoy it. Often it's tough to find the time to exercise, and it's tougher still to stick with something that you consider a bore or a chore. Today you've many options to choose from, so there's really no excuse.

And remember, there are many other reasons to exercise regularly. Exercise oxygenates your entire body, boosting circulation and giving you energy; helps you handle stress better and gives you a psychological lift and general sense of well-being; helps you live longer and healthier, since exercise is linked with reduction in heart disease, cancer, diabetes, and osteoporosis; improves sleep; helps normalize your weight; replaces flabby fat with firm, conditioned muscles; and helps you stay clear-headed and get more done for the time you put in—the time spent exercising is never time lost.

Strategy #4: Watch What You Eat

Your choice of foods has a central role to play in your immune power. Nutritionists recommend eating a diet that is balanced in carbohydrates, proteins, and fats and that contains adequate amounts of vitamins and minerals. You need to be wary of getting too much of some things and too little of others.

For example, eating too many sweets is bad for certain immune system cells called *neutrophils,* slowing down their ability to engulf and gobble up viruses. As little as 100 grams of sugar (the amount contained in two cans of soda) can cut neutrophil activity in half. Too much fat raises the risk of several diseases including cancer, which makes your immune system work harder and distract its energy from fighting off colds and flu. Foods and beverages containing caffeine and alcohol also reduce your immune power.

An immune-boosting diet is one that contains plenty of fresh fruits and vegetables (five to nine servings a day); whole grains such as brown rice or whole wheat (two to four servings per day); low-fat protein foods such as beans (one serving per day); and few if any servings of meat, dairy, and nuts. This eating pattern reduces the risk of many diseases besides infections, such as cancer, heart disease, diabetes, and more. Chapter 5 provides information about specific types of nutrients and guidelines to fine-tune your diet to strongly support your immune system. In Chapter 6 you'll find out how nutritional supplements can provide even more protection.

Strategy #5: Drink Up

A dry respiratory tract is an unhappy respiratory tract—and one that is more vulnerable to penetration by viruses. The mucous membrane lining your nose and throat needs a hydrated body to be moist enough to trap viruses and protect the cells. Sip liquids throughout the day so you're drinking a total of at least six to eight cups daily. Most natural medicine practitioners emphasize plain water—some advocate boiled water—and tea and/or diluted fruit juices. Avoid soda, coffee, and other caffeinated beverages, because these are diuretics and actually dry out your body. And go easy on the alcohol, which also slows down neutrophils.

Strategy #6: Get Humid

Low humidity impairs the immune responsivness of the mucous membranes in your nose, creating tiny fissures that let viruses penetrate to the cells below; it also has been found to impair your body's production of IgA, an immune component needed to fight cold viruses. Your respiratory tract also likes humid air, and viruses like it dry. No wonder colds and flu are more prevalent in winter, when the heat keeping our homes and offices comfortable dries the air. In summer, air conditioning can also suck moisture from the air. A Canadian study compared schools with 50 percent humidity with those that had 25 percent humidity. The higher-humidity schools had only half as many cold-related absences. So keep air moist in winter by opening the window, putting pans of water on radiators, or using a humidifier.

Strategy #7: Avoid Smoke and Pollution

Cigarette smoking is associated with a host of health problems. Smoking kills 300,000 Americans annually, and cuts ten to 15 years off life expectancy. Unlike an occasional glass of wine or beer, even light smoking is bad for you—each cigarette shortens life by five minutes. Smokers are ten times more likely to develop lung cancer than nonsmokers and two times more likely to develop heart disease. Cigarette smoke also is related to emphysema, chronic bronchitis, gum disease, and cancer of the mouth, throat, and bowel. It places an extra burden on the liver, which must detoxify the constituents of smoke such as cadmium, lead, and nicotine. Smoking depletes the body of several nutrients such as vitamin C, needed to combat infection. Smoking makes you look and feel older than your years. A recent study out of the Oregon Health Sciences University found that smoking made women age 65 and up feel older—they were less able to walk, climb stairs, or even get up out of a chair.

As if these weren't enough reasons to quit smoking or avoid secondhand smoke, several studies suggest that cigarettes increase susceptibility to colds. Children whose parents smoke are more likely to suffer from upper respiratory infections of all kinds. Air pollution also compromises the health of your respiratory system, so try to avoid breathing in car or bus fumes and other forms of pollution.

Strategy #8: Reduce Viral Exposure

The greater the number of viruses you are exposed to, and the greater the frequency of exposure, the higher your risk of becoming infected. So it's wise to take these simple measures.

• *Wash your hands often.* Get in the habit of washing your hands as soon as you get home or to work or after you have handled money to reduce the possibility of transferring a live virus from your hands to your nose or eyes. Try to educate children to wash their hands often too.

• *Keep your hands away from your face.* Try to be aware of how often you touch your nose or eyes and consciously reduce this tendency. If your eye itches, use a knuckle, not a fingertip. You don't need to pick your nose to give yourself the virus. According to cold researcher Jack Gwaltney, our hands find their way to our noses or eyes at least once every three hours, and a virus deposited at the base of your nose or eye can be inhaled or drain into the nasopharynx—the area of the throat from the back of the nose to the soft palate.

• *Avoid people with colds or flu as much as possible.* If you must share the same room, keep your distance. Airplane travel is particularly dangerous because of the close quarters and dry, virus-laden recirculated air.

• *Clean hard, nonporous surfaces.* Live viruses can cling to common everyday objects, waiting for you to pick them up with your hand. At work and home, use a disinfectant to cut down on the amount of virus that may settle on things you touch frequently, such as doorknobs, telephones, computer keyboards and accessories, door frames, countertops, major appliances, and toys.

• *Get the air moving.* Make sure there is adequate ventilation to reduce the concentration of viruses hovering in the air.

What About Vaccines?

Because the flu can be such a serious disease (epidemics killed half a million in the United States in 1918–1919; 34,000 in 1968), many medical doctors recommend routine flu vaccinations. Most natural medicine doctors do not recommend routine vaccinations; rather, they feel most people would be better off educating themselves about their immune systems and how to strengthen their resistance. However, because vaccines are made from a natural substance—the virus itself—and because they enhance your body's own immunity, natural medicine practitioners generally agree that flu shots are wise for people who are at high risk of complications or who may pass the illness on to many other people.

Vaccines are made from weakened or dead viruses and are quite specific to that one virus. Because there are over 200 cold viruses, it has been impossible to create a cold vaccine. However, since there are only a few active flu viruses every year, vaccines containing the most active viruses for that year are possible. A vaccine works in a similar fashion to being exposed to the actual virus—your body learns to recognize that particular bug and is able to fight it. If the flu viruses would stay the same from year to year, coming up with effective vaccines would be simple. But viruses change yearly. So, not only is there more than one flu virus, but the viruses that exist alter themselves constantly and sometimes dramatically. That means your immune system can't recognize most viruses that are floating around. Furthermore, infection with one particular flu virus protects you from reinfection with that one virus, but not others, and not even this year's version of the same virus! Similarly, last year's flu vaccination protects you against last year's viruses but not necessarily this year's. The Centers for Disease Control and Prevention (CDC) tracks changes in flu viruses each year and gathers worldwide information to help predict the optimal vaccine components for the following year. Typically, one or two of the three components are changed every year.

The CDC recommends annual flu shots for people who are at high risk of having a serious complication when they get the flu. This group includes:

- Everyone over the age of 65
- People, including children of any age, with certain

chronic health conditions, such as lung or heart disease or diabetes
- Health care providers who have frequent contact with people at high risk for serious flu complications
- Adults who provide child care
- Children who are on long-term aspirin therapy, because of the potential for Reye's syndrome
- Children who are in frequent contact with any of the above high-risk people

According to the CDC, flu vaccines are 70 to 90 percent effective in preventing flu among healthy adults. They may be less effective in elderly or chronically ill persons.

Two new "ouchless" forms of flu vaccine are being tested: A new type of influenza vaccine given in a nasal spray has been found to prevent flu in healthy young children. And a flu pill now being tested in adults has been able to prevent or cure influenza infections in animals. Both work by interfering with the reproduction of the virus.

CHAPTER FOUR

Taking Care of Yourself

Just because you're sick with a cold or flu doesn't mean you have to suffer. Using natural therapies to take care of yourself will help you relieve symptoms and get better as quickly as possible. In this chapter, you'll find eight general home-care strategies, followed by more specific advice for treating individual symptoms. For example, these simple, everyday practices help ease symptoms directly by using steam to unclog a stuffy nose, and indirectly by optimizing your natural cold-and-flu relief system—your immunity. And while you'll probably be able to take care of yourself at home, it's important to understand the warning signs that indicate professional care is in order. Therefore this chapter gives you safety guidelines and tips on how to find a qualified natural medicine practitioner.

Eight Strategies for Treating Colds and Flu

A cold usually lasts from four to seven days; influenza lasts one week to ten days. Although there's no cure for either, there's plenty you can do to lessen the suffering and possibly shorten the duration as well. Some natural medicine practitioners feel the common cold or flu is nature's way of telling us to slow down and take it easy—an early-warning sign that we're depleting our defenses. In fact, many also hesitate to recommend medicine of any kind, even herbs or homeopathic medicine, because the condition is so benign it's better to just rest, blow our noses, drink fluids, and let our immune systems do their job.

Self-Care Strategy #1: Rest

Make sure you take time out to rest during the illness to keep your immune system on the ball. You don't necessarily have to stay in bed during a cold, but do take it easy so you don't tax your reserves of energy, which could be put to better use fighting the infection. The energy used to fight a cold or flu has been compared to hard physical labor—so it's no wonder you feel tired while you're sick. During a flu you may feel so exhausted you have no choice but to stay in bed. Furthermore, staying home from work or school during your most contagious days (when symptoms are just beginning and are at their height) reduces the number of people exposed to your particular bug and, in the long run, reduces sick days and increases productivity in general. Despite the fatigue brought on by illness, some people may have trouble sleeping because of discomfort. If this is the case, try taking an herbal or homeopathic remedy to help you fall asleep and stay asleep.

As you feel better, slowly increase your activity, beginning with perhaps a few stretches to get out the kinks that may settle in your back and joints from inactivity. Once you are on the mend, you can resume your exercise program gradually. The general rule is: Once you feel well enough to exercise, wait one more day. Another guideline is to take a "neck check." If your symptoms are above the neck, you probably have a mild cold—and that gives you the green light to keep up your usual exercise routine. (But stop if you begin to feel worse.) A fever or symptoms below the neck means your body is working hard enough and your most strenuous exercise should be sipping hot tea.

Self-Care Strategy #2: Drink Up

Drink plenty of fluids, such as water or fruit juices diluted with water, to help keep mucus flowing and replace fluid lost through sweating. Hot bland liquids may be particularly comforting and loosen phlegm, whereas cold liquids may worsen congestion by slowing down the flow of nasal mucus. Hot soups and hot teas (see Chapters 3 and 5) are a tasty way to get more fluid into your body, and they have specific therapeutic properties as well. Usually, eight ounces of liquid every two hours is recommended.

Self-Care Strategy #3: Clear Pathways

Blow your nose rather than sniffling and swallowing mucus to rid your system of the virus. The safest way to blow is to clear one nostril and then the other, because doing so puts less air pressure on your respiratory system and ear canal. Be sure to cough up any phlegm frequently. Teach young children how to do this; in infants, use a small bulb syringe to evacuate mucus from the nose. Salt water, or saline, nasal sprays are available commercially, but you can easily make your own saline solution. Mix 1/3 teaspoon noniodized table salt and a pinch of baking soda with 1 cup lukewarm filtered or bottled water (nonchlorinated). Place in a clean spray bottle. Pinch one nostril closed and spray the other nostril while inhaling; then repeat with the other nostril. Do this as often as you need to relieve a clogged-up nose. If this does not provide enough relief, you may want to use the same salt solution for the nasal wash technique (see "Sinusitis," page 47), which is a more intense and more effective method.

Self-Care Strategy #4: Moisturize

Keep the air moist with a humidifier or vaporizer; or inhale steam from a bowl of hot water (make a hood by draping a towel over your head) to further loosen mucus and make breathing easier. However, avoid extreme heat, such as steam baths and saunas, and extreme cold as well. The May 18, 1997, issue of *Consumer Reports* evaluates humidifiers and gives guidelines on how to choose one. They rated the best tabletop model to be the Duracraft DH-904 and best console models the Toastmaster 3435 and the Emerson HD14W1. (For the worksheet that helps you gauge your individual humidification needs, send a stamped, self-addressed envelope to Consumer Reports, Box DY, 101 Truman Avenue, Yonkers, NY 10703-1057.)

A note of caution: there is no perfect type of humidifier. Steam-mist models (also called "vaporizers") can cause scalding if you tip them over or get too close to the mist. Evaporative models, which are the most common, can be a breeding ground for mold and bacteria and thus require frequent cleaning. Be sure your humidifier has a humidistat so you can check that the relative humidity stays between 30 and 60 percent, which is considered to be optimum. Less than that is ineffective, and more than that can corrode metal, rot wood, and encourage the growth of mold, mildew, mites, and other organisms that aggravate allergies.

Self-Care Strategy #5: Eat Lightly

Eat a light diet of bland, well-cooked food. You've probably heard the old adage about starving a cold and feeding a fever and been confused by it. That's because it has been corrupted from the original sage advice, "If you feed a cold, you will have to starve a fever." Originally attributed to Hippocrates, it contains a kernel of truth: If you tax your body with food during a cold, you will worsen and eventually get a fever. The main point is that eating during an infection is not wise. Fasting or eating very lightly eases the load on the body. Eliminate the hard-to-digest foods, so you can devote your energy to healing, not to digesting and dealing with toxins in food. Many natural health practitioners advise you to avoid dairy products because they produce mucus. You'll find information about the specific therapeutic effects of particular foods in Chapter 5.

Self-Care Strategy #6: Protect Others

Although you may subscribe to the theory that misery loves company, there's a lot you can do to reduce the likelihood of spreading your cold or flu to others. Colds are most contagious during the first three days of symptoms. Cover your mouth and nose when you cough and sneeze to reduce virus-laden droplets spraying through the air. Wash your hands often with plenty of soap and water to lessen the possibility of your contaminated hands passing the virus to others by hand-to-hand contact or hand-to-object-to-hand contact. Use disposable tissues; cloth handkerchiefs can harbor live viruses for several hours and can recontaminate your fingers. Disinfect surfaces that you come into contact with and that others may touch later, such as telephones and doorknobs. Stay away from healthy people, particularly if you have the flu; flu viruses spread more easily through the air than do cold viruses. And don't suppress a sneeze—sneezing forces air through your nose and mouth at about 100 miles an hour, enough to damage your eardrum if redirected to your Eustachian tube.

Self-Care Strategy #7: Don't Smoke

Many people who smoke automatically kick the habit during an illness. This makes sense—and not just because smoking further irritates the throat and lungs. When you inhale smoke (yours or someone else's), it paralyzes the tiny hairs that sweep out pathogens and mucus, slowing recovery time.

Self-Care Strategy #8: Use Natural Medicine

Consider using the specific natural therapies presented in the later chapters of this book. They have a synergistic effect when used along with these basic self-care practices, so they will provide additional symptom relief and boost your immune power.

Home Care to Ease Specific Symptoms

In addition to the general measures just given, you may find the following helpful in soothing specific symptoms such as sore throat, cough, laryngitis, and fever as well as complications such as sinusitis and earache. Don't forget to turn to the chapters on individual natural therapies, where you'll find even more powerful remedies for treating these symptoms.

Sore Throat, Cough, or Laryngitis

A sore throat can be the most painful symptom of a cold or flu. Coughing is a reflex that acts as a defense mechanism. An irritation or obstruction in one of the breathing tubes triggers the mechanism, which creates a strong upward rush of air. This explosive movement forces the irritating or obstructing material out of the tube. Natural home care therapy does not try to suppress the coughing reflex since it represents the body's best efforts to expel something harmful—such as viruses, bacteria, or irritants—from breathing passages.

Laryngitis is an inflammation of the mucous membrane lining the voice box (larynx) plus a swelling of the vocal cords, which causes hoarseness or loss of voice. The following should help your cough be more effective, while soothing the throat and minimizing unnecessary coughing:

- Stop smoking, if you smoke.
- Drink plenty of fluids to lubricate the throat.
- Try to cough up any phlegm.
- Increase the humidity of the air in the room with a humidifier or vaporizer, or inhale steam from a vaporizer or bowl of heated water. This helps lubricate the throat, soothe an inflamed larynx and encourage healing, and thin the mucus so it is easier to expel.
- Gargling with warm salt water (¼ teaspoon noniodized salt dissolved in 1 cup chlorine-free water) helps soothe a sore throat, reduce inflammation, and flush away viruses and bacteria as well as mucus and postnasal drip secretions which could irritate your throat and trigger a cough.
- Rest the throat and voice as much as possible.

Seek Medical Care If . . . the pain is severe; swallowing is very difficult or painful; there is a lot of saliva and drooling; there is difficulty breathing; laryngitis lasts more than seven days; the sore throat is accompanied by fever and doesn't improve in 48 hours with home care.

Fever

Fever, though it may be uncomfortable, is a positive sign that your body is defending itself from infection and has many beneficial functions. It speeds the metabolism so more blood, oxygen, and nutrients can reach tissues. Waste products such as dead cells and dead viruses are carried away more quickly. The extra heat slows down the invading organism and makes it more vulnerable to the germ-fighting components of your immune system.

This powerful, natural defense mechanism usually is not a cause for concern, and in most cases it should be left alone to do its job during an acute illness. The following should make you feel more comfortable and support the healing efforts of the body:

- Learn how to take a temperature to confirm and evaluate the severity of a fever. Oral thermometers work best for most individuals; rectal or axillary (armpit) thermometers work best in young children.
- Protect yourself from drafts and make sure you don't become chilled.
- Rest combats the exhaustion fever sometimes brings, and drinking plenty of liquids replaces the fluids lost through sweating.
- Have someone give you a sponge bath with tepid water for about 20 minutes to relieve the fever. As the water evaporates, it cools the skin and the blood flowing close to the surface, bringing the overall temperature down. Be careful of drafts during the procedure and pat dry when finished.
- Sometimes just sponging the face and neck—and per-

haps one limb at a time—increases comfort considerably.

- To make the bath more effective by promoting sweating, you may add yarrow tea to the water. Make a potent yarrow tea by adding 3 tablespoons herb to 2 cups boiling water. Let steep for 20 minutes, strain, and dilute with another 2 cups boiling water and add it to the bathwater. The yarrow increases circulation to the skin surface and acts as an anti-inflammatory.

NEVER give aspirin to a child who has fever that may be due to viral infection, as aspirin increases the risk of a serious liver and brain disease known as Reye's syndrome.

Seek Medical Care If . . . a baby under six months of age has a fever; an older baby has had a fever for more than 24 hours that hasn't responded to homeopathic home care or remedies; the fever is over 105 degrees F in a person of any age; a child has had a (fever-related) seizure during either a past or current illness; there are signs of dehydration.

Canker Sores and Cold Sores

Canker or cold sores can erupt when you are under any kind of stress, such as a cold or flu. People often confuse canker sores and cold sores and use the terms interchangeably. However, it is important to decide which condition you have, because cold sores (herpes) are contagious, while canker sores are not.

A *canker sore* is an ulcer of the mouth. The irregularly shaped sores may occur on the tongue, on the inside of the cheeks, or on the insides of the lips. Canker sores look as if the tissue has been burned, with a red ring surrounding a white circular sore. A canker sore forms when the body is unable to retain the integrity of the mucous membrane lining of the mouth.

Cold sores (also known as "fever blisters") often appear around the mouth and lips and are outward signs that the body is carrying the Type 1 herpes simplex virus. After the initial outbreak—about three to six days after infection—the herpes simplex virus normally lies dormant until there is some form of stress to throw the body off-balance. Cold sores look like tiny blisters (vesicles) in the midst of red, inflamed skin. The vesicles contain a clear liquid that may turn into pus. The vesicles open, leaving a sore that eventually heals. Type 2 herpes simplex virus causes genital sores, which also may resurface during a stress such as cold or flu.

If your cold or flu triggers these sores, keep the following in mind:

- Keep sores clean and dry by gently washing with mild soap and water twice a day.
- Do not kiss other people while you have cold sores; doing so can spread the herpes virus. Use separate towels until the sores are completely healed.
- Don't squeeze the blisters.
- Keep sun exposure to a minimum if you have cold sores.
- Rinse your mouth several times a day with a mouthwash made of 1 tablespoon sea salt dissolved in ½ cup warm water.
- Avoid toothpaste containing the detergent sodium lauryl sulfate (SLS) if you get canker sores. In a small study, it was found that people who used SLS-free toothpaste for three months had 70 percent fewer mouth sores.

Seek Medical Care If . . . sores recur often or are very severe; if the skin around the eyes is affected; if sores become infected; and if you see no improvement after five to seven days of natural medicine treatment. Seek immediate medical care if the eye becomes inflamed or painful. A person with an active infection should cover the blisters and wash his or her hands thoroughly before touching someone who is particularly vulnerable, such as children, the elderly, a person with AIDS, or receiving chemotherapy.

Sinusitis

Sinuses are cavities in your skull—the open spaces above the eyes, within the nose, and inside the cheekbones (See Figure 4.1). Your sinuses lighten the weight of the bone that houses your brain. It is believed they also protect your lungs by humidifying the air, regulating air temperature, and filtering out viruses, bacteria, and particles that might cause problems.

Sinusitis is a swelling of these cavities. The problem often starts with the common cold, which causes the mucous membrane lining the sinus to become swollen. This blocks off the opening leading from the sinus to the nose. The virus also can paralyze the cilia—tiny hairs lining the respiratory tract that act as natural brooms. When they cease their constant sweeping motion, mucus stops flowing freely and becomes a breeding ground for bacteria. When the sinuses become overwhelmed with a bacterial infection, symptoms worsen and there may be a pus-filled discharge from the nose.

Each year 35 million Americans develop sinus infections, according to the American Academy of Otolaryngology. Sinusitis frequently is mistaken for a cold, because one often follows the other and symptoms are similar. If you catch a cold that persists or worsens after

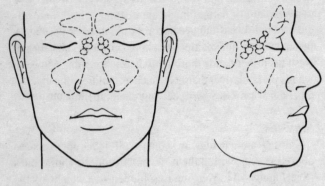

Figure 4.1

seven to ten days, it is probably a sinus infection. Symptoms are mainly a feeling of fullness or congestion in the nose and entire head, head or facial pain (including a dull ache above, between, and behind the eyes, in the forehead, and in the cheeks or upper teeth—depending on the sinus cavities infected), dizziness or lightheadedness, thick green/yellow nasal mucus or postnasal drip, bad breath, and extreme fatigue. Sinusitis may be mild or severe, acute, chronic, or recurring. Sinusitis may affect only one side of the head, or both. Untreated, symptoms may last for two or more weeks and sometimes several months.

Sinusitis is a condition that can become chronic and permanently weaken the sinuses. If you have a sinus problem, natural medicine offers hope and an alternative to antibiotics. (Half of sinus infections are bacterial in nature.) Following the natural approaches in this book may help shorten the duration and lessen the severity of your cold symptoms, help relieve sinus symptoms should they occur, and improve your overall resistance to colds and sinus infections.

If your cold is accompanied by sinus pain, the following measures will make you more comfortable and speed healing.

- Take it easy and get rest, especially if the sinusitis is severe.
- Use a vaporizer, humidifier, or bowl of steaming water to loosen mucus and relieve sinus congestion. Wet, hot compresses applied to the painful area also may be soothing.
- Drink plenty of fluids to help liquefy mucus secretions.
- To reduce swelling of the nasal passages and rinse away mucus, use a nasal wash several times a day. (See Figure 4.2.) Make a saline solution (salt water) by dissolving ⅓ teaspoon noniodized table salt and a pinch baking soda in 1 cup filtered or bottled water. Put the saline solution in a rubber ear syringe (available in most drugstores), an eye dropper, or a "neti pot" (a device used in yoga practice and available in many health food stores). Using ½ cup solution for each nostril, stand leaning with your head over a sink or basin. Pinch one nostril closed and insert the tip of whatever device you are using in the other nostril. Pinch that nostril closed around the tip and gently squeeze the solution into your nose. The solution will come out both nostrils and probably your mouth. You may try this without pinching the nostrils, but doing so may not remove as much mucus. An alternate method is to pour the solution into the palm of your

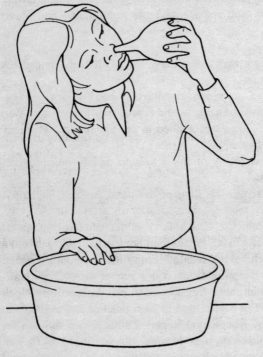

Figure 4.2

hand and sniff it. Be sure to blow your nose thoroughly after doing a nasal wash.

Seek Medical Care If . . . the sinus pain is severe, there is high fever or a smelly discharge, or if an infection doesn't improve with home care in 48 hours.

Ear Infection

Ear infection is a complication of upper respiratory infection and can happen at any age but occurs most often in children. In fact, it is the most common complication in children and is responsible for an estimated 25 percent of all visits to pediatricians. *Otitis media* is the term used for an infection of the middle ear, the space behind the eardrum. Colds and allergies often lay the groundwork for middle ear infections by narrowing the Eustachian tube that leads from the middle ear to the nasal passages (See Figure 4.3). The ear fluids that normally drain through the tube into the throat accumulate in this space, causing blockage and a comfortable environment for bacterial growth. Young children are particularly vulnerable because their tubes are so small and short. In children, symptoms are ear pain, fever, crying and fussiness, pulling the ears, restless sleep, and temporary hearing loss. The eardrum may rupture and allow a discharge to flow out. Since most ear infections are bacterial, the standard conventional treatment is antibiotics. However, most ear infections go away without antibiotic treatment, especially if you follow the home care measures below; herbal and homeopathic remedies also can help you avoid antibiotics.

- Learn to evaluate and diagnose ear infections. Ask your health care professional to show you how to use

an *otoscope* (available at pharmacies) to examine the ears of family members.
- As with any infection, rest helps the healing process.
- Consuming plenty of fluids helps keep secretions fluid and replaces water lost through perspiration.
- Moist heat, much as a hot towel or washcloth, or a hot water bottle may soothe pain. Some people find cold relieves pain.
- Avoid inserting objects to clean out stopped-up or pus-filled ears. This only drives the material in farther and may puncture the eardrum.
- Flush out packed-in wax with a syringe filled with warm water or hydrogen peroxide diluted with 4 parts water.

Seek Medical Care If . . . home care measures fail to improve an earache within 24 hours in a young child, or in two to three days in an older child or adult. Get medical care if there is extreme weakness, severe pain, or stiff neck; if there is any swelling, redness, or pain behind the ear; if there is fever accompanied by a profuse ear discharge; or if there is hearing loss that extends beyond two weeks. Have the ear examined by your physician three weeks after successful home care treatment to make sure the healing is complete.

Finding a Qualified Health Care Professional

You may want to consult a professional particularly if you have severe symptoms, if you have given self-care a try but symptoms haven't improved or have gotten worse, or if you get colds and flu frequently, indicating a stressed-out immune system.

Unfortunately, there is no nationally recognized stan-

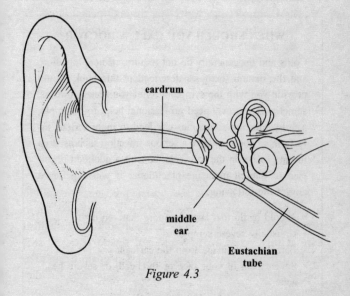

Figure 4.3

dard degree, licensing procedure, or certification for practitioners of natural approaches, so finding a reputable practitioner can be a challenge. However, there are more and more certifying programs and boards for some practices such as homeopathy and herbal therapy. Ask your physician or other trusted health care professional for a referral, or ask a friend or relative who has gotten good results. Alternatively, you can refer to Appendix A, ''Resources,'' and contact the appropriate professional associations for lists of qualified individuals in your area.

A *naturopathic doctor* (N.D.) will offer the most choices in types of natural medicine. Naturopathic train-

---

WHEN SHOULD YOU CALL A DOCTOR?

Colds and flu generally do not require medical attention, and the natural therapies described in this book should provide you with the symptom relief you seek. However, sometimes you may need professional help; for example, a mild infection sometimes can lead to more serious infection, or you may have a serious infection such as strep throat. To be on the safe side, consult a qualified physician or natural medicine practitioner if you experience any of the following:

- A cold or flu that lasts for more than ten days
- Unusually severe symptoms
- Earache or drainage from the ear canal
- Severe pain in your face or forehead, or severe headache
- Temperature above 102 degrees F
- Shortness of breath or wheezing
- Hoarseness, sore throat, or cough that doesn't go away
- Chest pain
- Convulsions, delirium
- Extreme weakness
- A stiff neck
- Sudden unexpected vomiting
- Light-colored stools

and remember . . .

If you are presently taking medication, are pregnant or nursing, are over the age of 70 or under the age of ten, or are under medical treatment for a specific medical condition, it is essential to consult your doctor before administering any natural medicine.

ing involves completion of four years of naturopathic medical school, which includes extensive understanding of conventional physiology and pathology but is based on natural medicines such as nutrition, herbs, stress management, and massage or physical manipulation. Students are supervised in their training clinics but have no hospital training and may not prescribe medicines. Naturopaths take a qualifying exam in homeopathy that confers a Diplomat status of the Homeopathic Academy of Naturopathic Physicians (D.H.A.N.P.). As of this writing, naturopaths are licensed in a number of states: Alaska, Arizona, Connecticut, District of Columbia, Florida, Hawaii, Idaho, Montana, North Carolina, Oregon, Utah, and Washington. In several other states legislation is pending to license naturopaths.

There are 1,500 licensed or licensable naturopaths in the United States, with thousands more in other states that do not confer licenses. The American Holistic Medical Association has 600 members, and about 10,000 other M.D.'s or D.O.'s (doctors of osteopathy) use some holistic approaches. Depending on where you live, you may not have a tremendous choice in natural health practitioners. However, be sure to ask about their credentials. Find out:

- Where the practitioner studied and for how long.
- How long the practitioner has been in practice: Ask specifically how much of his or her time has been devoted exclusively to natural medicine. Obviously,

the more experienced practitioner is usually more skilled.

- If he or she belongs to the American Association of Naturopathic Physicians or the American Holistic Medical Association.

CHAPTER FIVE

Food as Medicine

This chapter will show you how food can keep you healthy and help you recover from an illness. Using food as medicine has a long history—in fact, food was probably the first basic form of medicine available. In terms of understanding the healing power of food, we've come a long way from the simple admonishment to "eat your vegetables." Of course, eating vegetables is still a good idea—in fact, eating more fresh fruits and vegetables is one of the key changes Americans need to make in their diet to lower risk of many diseases from colds to cancer. But now scientists have a better understanding as to why plant foods and other foods are such potent health-builders, and you can use this knowledge in your everyday life.

This chapter begins with how a good diet can be used as a preventive measure. First you'll find a concise guide to better eating and a summary description of the nutrients you need to get every day. You'll also find a guide to using common herbs and spices that are delicious as well as immune-enhancing. Next comes a primer on using food as therapy—single foods like tea, simple nourishing recipes, and still more herbs and spices known for their recuperative powers. Finally this chapter looks at the role food allergies can play and how fasting is a healing tool you may want to consider.

Food as Preventive Medicine

While research is scanty on how to use food to prevent colds and flu specifically, an overwhelming amount of evidence supports food as a general immune-enhancer. An immune-enhancing eating pattern consists of a variety of foods and emphasizes fresh fruits, vegetables, and whole grains that are high in vitamins and minerals; a moderate amount of protein foods; and a modest amount of fat with the emphasis on the right kinds of fats. This way of eating not only helps keep your immune system humming; it also improves your health generally and may decrease your risk of serious diseases, such as heart disease and cancer.

What's Wrong with the Way You're Eating?

The abbreviation for the Standard American Diet is SAD, and the way most Americans eat certainly is "sad." Numerous surveys show that the average diet is too low in nourishing vitamins, minerals, and fiber, and too high in fat, protein, and refined starches and sugars. The RDAs (Recommended Dietary Allowances), established by the National Academy of Sciences, defines the levels of the essential vitamins and minerals adequate to prevent deficiency diseases. According to a recent U.S. Department of Agriculture survey, which studied the three-day food intake of 21,500 people, *not one single person* consumed 100 percent of the RDA for the ten nutrients included in the survey. In addition, research suggests that perhaps one-quarter of Americans are not getting balanced amounts of essential fatty acids. (These are a "good" component of fat that are discussed in greater detail later in this chapter.) As you'll see in the next chapter, even the RDAs may be too low for optimum health, and you may wish to augment your diet with nutritional supplements.

Better Eating Guidelines

Although there's evidence that nutritional supplements can be both preventive and therapeutic, even supplement advocates recommend that food be the foundation for better health and strengthened immunity.

In revamping your eating patterns, use the following three basic principles as your guide.

- Emphasize whole, fresh foods.
- Limit fatty foods.
- Limit animal products.

To help you create healthy eating habits, refer to the following table of daily eating guidelines. It gives you a general idea of the food groups and the amount you should consume each day.

DAILY EATING GUIDELINES

Low-Starch Vegetables

3–4 cups low-starch vegetables such as broccoli, carrots, spinach, lettuce, onions, celery, string beans, artichoke, summer squash, endive, cabbage, cucumbers, asparagus, chard, peppers, parsley, sprouts, tomatoes. (Include 1 cup high-calcium leafy greens such as collards, kale, dandelion and turnip greens, or bok choy.)

Starchy Vegetables
1–2 servings (½ cup each) potatoes, yams, sweet potatoes, parsnips, winter squash, or turnips

Whole Grains
1–2 slices whole-grain bread, plus at least 2 cups brown rice, oats, corn, millet, barley, buckwheat, amaranth, quinoa, wheat, triticale, or rye

Fresh Fruit
1–3 per day

Beans
1 or more ½-cup servings: split peas, lentils, kidney beans, navy beans, chickpeas, aduki beans, black beans, white beans, mung or soy beans, tofu

Meat, Fish, Poultry
None, or limit to one 4–5 ounce serving per day or less; fish is preferable; fresh lean meats such as turkey or chicken in moderation

Dairy
0–3 servings; 1 serving is 1 cup low-fat or fat-free milk or yogurt; ½ cup cottage cheese; 1 ounce cheese

Essential Fats
2–3 teaspoons unrefined vegetable oils of flax seed, safflower, or sesame. Refrigerate all oils.

Other Oils
Olive oil does not have essential fatty acids but is stable and, unlike polyunsaturated oil, is not damaged by heat.

Nuts and Seeds

A small amount of fresh, unsalted nuts and seeds (⅛–¼ cup) or nut butter if desired. Home-roasted sunflower, sesame, or pumpkin seeds are a delicious snack or garnish.

Water

At least eight 8-ounce glasses; purified or spring water is preferred.

Health-Building Nutrients to Eat Every Day

The guidelines above tell you *what* you should eat. In this section, you'll find out *why* you should eat that way. This type of eating pattern is most likely to supply you with the following nutrients—nutrients you need to eat every day in order to make sure you are feeding your immune system and other related body systems. Be aware that even if you follow these guidelines faithfully, it's still very difficult to get everything you need through just food alone. You may want to follow the nutritional supplement program provided in Chapter 6 to help reach and maintain optimum health.

THE ANTIOXIDANTS

Free radicals are unstable molecules that form when fats and other substances combine with oxygen in the body. We're exposed to free radicals from indoor and outdoor air pollution, pollutants in our food and water, alcohol, drugs, cigarette smoke, and radiation. Our bodies also produce them as by-products of normal metabolism; thus free radicals are needed for survival. However, they are dangerous when there are too many of them and they overload our system. Free radicals can attack any part of the cell—including the genetic material in the nucleus, cell walls, and particularly those parts that contain polyunsaturated fatty acids (PUFAs). When unchecked, free radicals generate more free radicals, and this chain reaction may cause cells to die, malfunction, or become cancerous; tissues and organs may be damaged. Your immune system, whose job it is to clean up and remove damaged cells, suddenly is overburdened. Free radicals may even damage the organs of the immune system. Free-radical damage, also called oxidation, is what causes metal to rust, rubber to turn brittle, butter to turn rancid, and paintings to deteriorate. In the human body it has been associated with immune problems and many diseases and conditions, including premature aging and death, cardiovascular disease, many types of cancer, diabetes, cataracts and other degenerative eye problems, arthritis, and possibly osteoporosis.

Nature, in its wisdom, designed our bodies to produce antioxidant enzymes that keep free radicals under control. Luckily for us several vitamins and minerals also act as antioxidants. So it stands to reason that keeping an optimum level of these nutrients in the body may cut down on the number of colds and flu experienced.

VITAMINS

Vitamins are organic compounds—in other words, they occur naturally in plants and animals. They are used most often as coenzymes, which means they help activate the chemical reactions our bodies produce to stay alive. Breathing, blinking, reading, running, digesting, fighting viruses—enzymes and vitamin coenzymes are needed for our every action and reaction. Fresh fruits and vegetables and whole grains are rich sources of vitamins.

In addition to their coenzyme status, vitamins have many other specific functions; many of them are related to immune function.

Vitamin A and its precursor, beta-carotene, are also antioxidants and stimulate production of antibodies, T-cells, and natural killer cells (which fight cancer). Vitamin A also maintains epithelial cells and mucous membranes—physical barriers that serve as your first line of defense against invasion by harmful viruses.

B-complex vitamins are used by your body to produce immune system components: T-cells, B-cells, antibodies, and other immune-system proteins. All the B-vitamins—B-1 (thiamin), B-2 (riboflavin), B-3 (niacin), B-6 (pyridoxine), B-12 (cobalamin), folic acid, pantothenic acid, biotin, choline, inositol, and PABA (para-aminobenzoic acid) work together in the body and are needed for many functions.

Vitamin C is an antioxidant. It stimulates white blood cells, which scavenge and dissolve viruses and other invaders, promotes production of interferon, which stimulates immune activity, and blocks the effects of a stress hormone that dampens immune activity.

Vitamin E is also a potent antioxidant; in addition, it has been shown to enhance the activity of white cells and improve resistance to disease.

MINERALS

Unlike vitamins, minerals are not organic—they are inorganic, meaning they are not produced by plants or animals. However, they too function as coenzymes and thus are crucial to the maintenance of all body processes. The major minerals needed by the body are calcium, magnesium, phosphorus, manganese, zinc, iron, copper, chromium, selenium, iodine, potassium, and boron. Some minerals have specific immune-enhancing or supporting effects, in particular zinc and selenium. As is the case with vitamins, fresh fruits and vegetables and whole grains are the best sources for minerals, provided the soil they are grown in contains adequate minerals.

FLAVONOIDS AND OTHER PHYTONUTRIENTS

Probably many other food components, only some of which have been discovered, let alone studied, support immune function. An important group is called *flavonoids*. Flavonoids are not-quite vitamins that are found in many vegetables, fruits, and grains, often in the company of vitamin C. Foods especially rich in flavonoids include the most colorful fruits and vegetables—the more colorful and the deeper the color, the better: apricots, beets, blueberries, cherries, parsley, peaches, plums, raspberries, red grapes, rhubarb, spinach, and strawberries. They also are found in many herbs, green tea, and garlic, along with other *phytonutrients* or *phytochemicals* (*phyto* means "plant") that are antioxidants and stimulate enzymes and thus have remarkable healing and health-maintaining powers. Among their many abilities, flavonoids are antioxidants and have antiviral effects.

VITAMINS AND MINERALS—WHAT THEY DO AND WHERE TO FIND THEM

Nutrient	Major Uses	Food Sources
	Fat-Soluble Vitamins	
Vitamin A and Beta-carotene	Antioxidant	Fish liver oils, animal livers, green and yellow fruits and vegetables
	Prevents night blindness and other eye problems	
	May be useful for acne and other skin disorders	
	Enhances immunity	
	Cancer prevention	

Nutrient	Major Uses	Food Sources
	May heal gastrointestinal ulcers	
	Protects against pollution	
	Needed for epithelial tissue maintenance and repair	
Vitamin D	Required for calcium and phosphorus absorption and utilization	Fish liver oils, fatty saltwater fish, vitamin D-fortified dairy products, eggs
	Prevention and treatment of osteoporosis	
	Enhances immunity	
Vitamin E	Antioxidant	Cold-pressed vegetable oils, whole grains, nuts, dark-green leafy vegetables, legumes
	Cancer prevention	
	Cardiovascular disease prevention	
	Improves circulation	
	Tissue repair	
	May prevent age spots	
	Useful in treating fibrocystic breasts	
	Useful in treating PMS	
Vitamin K	Needed for blood clotting	Green leafy vegetables
	May play a role in bone formation	
	May prevent osteoporosis	

Nutrient	Major Uses	Food Sources
	Water-Soluble Vitamins	
Biotin	Needed for metabolism of protein, fats, and carbohydrates	Meat, cooked egg yolk, yeast, poultry, milk, saltwater fish, soybeans, whole grains
	Not enough data available, but deficiencies may be implicated in high serum cholesterol, seborrheic dermatitis, and certain nervous system disorders	
Choline and Inositol	Involved in metabolism of fat and cholesterol, and absorption and utilization of fat	Egg yolk, whole grains, vegetables, organ meats, fruits, milk
	Choline makes an important brain neurotransmitter	
Folic acid	Works closely with B-12	Beef, lamb, pork, chicken liver, whole wheat, bran, green leafy vegetables, yeast
	Involved in protein metabolism	
	Needed for healthy cell division and replication	
	Prevention and treatment of folic acid anemia	
	Stress may increase need	
	May be useful for depression and anxiety	
	May be useful in treating cervical dysplasia	
	Oral contraceptives may increase need	

Nutrient	Major Uses	Food Sources
PABA	Needed for protein metabolism Needed for folic acid metabolism Used topically as a sunscreen	Liver, kidney, whole grains, molasses
Pantothenic acid	Needed in fat, protein, and carbohydrate metabolism Needed for synthesis of hormones and cholesterol Needed for red blood cell production Needed for nerve transmission Vital for healthy function of the adrenal glands May be useful for joint inflammation May be useful for depression and anxiety	Eggs, saltwater fish, pork, beef, milk, whole wheat, beans, fresh vegetables
Vitamin B Complex B-1 (thiamin); B-2 (riboflavin); B-3 (niacin, niacinamide); B-6 (pyridoxine)	Maintains healthy nerves, skin, eyes, hair, liver, mouth, muscle tone in gastrointestinal tract B vitamins are coenzymes involved in energy production Emotional or physical stress increases need May be useful for depression or anxiety	Unrefined whole grains, liver, green leafy vegetables, fish, poultry, eggs, meat, nuts, beans

Nutrient	Major Uses	Food Sources
Vitamin B-12 (cobalamin)	Needed for fat and carbohydrate metabolism Prevention and treatment of B-12 anemia Maintains proper nervous system function May be useful for anxiety and depression	Kidney, liver, egg, herring, mackerel, milk, cheese, tofu, seafood
Vitamin C (ascorbic acid)	Growth and repair of tissues May reduce cholesterol Antioxidant Cancer prevention Enhances immunity Stress increases requirement May reduce high blood pressure May prevent atherosclerosis Protects against pollution	Green vegetables, berries, citrus fruit
Boron	Prevents bone loss May enhance bone density	Fruits, vegetables
Calcium	Needed for healthy bones and teeth Needed for nerve transmission Used for muscle function May lower blood pressure Osteoporosis prevention	Dairy foods, green leafy vegetables, salmon, sardines, seafood

Nutrient	Major Uses	Food Sources
Chromium	Required for glucose metabolism May prevent diabetes May reduce cholesterol	Brewer's yeast, beer, meat, cheese, whole grains
Copper	Involved in blood formation Needed for healthy nerves Needed for taste sensitivity Used in energy production Needed for healthy bone development	Widely distributed in foods, also derived from copper cookware and plumbing
Iodine	Needed for healthy thyroid gland Prevents goiter	Iodized salts, seafood, kelp, saltwater fish
Iron	Vital for blood formation Needed for energy production Required for healthy immune system	Meat, poultry, fish, liver, eggs, green leafy vegetables, whole-grain or enriched breads and cereals
Magnesium	Needed for healthy bones Involved in nerve transmission Needed for muscle function Used in energy formation	Widely distributed in foods, especially dairy foods,

Nutrient	Major Uses	Food Sources
	Needed for healthy blood vessels	meat, fish, seafood
	May lower blood pressure	
Manganese	Needed for protein and fat metabolism	Nuts, seeds, whole grains, avocado, seaweed
	Used in energy formation	
	Required for normal bone growth and reproduction	
	Needed for healthy nerves	
	Needed for healthy blood sugar regulation	
	Needed for healthy immune system	
Phosphorus	Necessary for healthy bones	Available in most foods; sodas can be very high
	Needed for production of energy	
	Used as a buffering agent	
	Needed for utilization of protein, fats, and carbohydrates	
Potassium	May lower blood pressure	Dairy foods, meat, poultry, fish, fruit, legumes, whole grains, vegetables
	Needed for energy storage	
	Needed for nerve transmission, muscle contraction, and hormone secretion	
Selenium	Cancer prevention	Depending on soil content,
	Heart disease prevention	

Nutrient	Major Uses	Food Sources
		may be in grains and meat
Zinc	Needed for wound healing Maintains taste and smell acuity Needed for healthy immune system Protects liver from chemical damage	Oysters, fish, seafood, meats, poultry, whole grains, legumes
Coenzyme Q_{10} (CoQ)	Cell energy and metabolism Prevents cell damage May be useful in cardiovascular diseases such as angina, congestive heart failure, arrhythmia, and high blood pressure May protect heart muscle and promote faster recovery from heart attack and heart surgery	None
Flavonoids	Antioxidant May lower cholesterol May prevent cardiovascular disease May inhibit cancer Needed to maintain healthy blood vessels Helps fight viral infections	Fruits, vegetables, grains, nuts, seeds, soybeans, tea, coffee, wine

Nutrient	Major Uses	Food Sources
Garlic	May lower blood pressure	Garlic
	May enhance immune system	
	May prevent heart disease	
	May lower triglycerides	
	May lower cholesterol	
	Antibacterial, antiviral, antifungal	
	Prevents excess blood clotting	
	May prevent cancer	
	Antioxidant	
Omega-3	Prevents heart disease	Cold-water fish
	May lower blood pressure	
	May lower triglycerides	
	May lower cholesterol	
	Prevents excess blood clotting	
	May relieve inflammatory and allergic reactions	
	May inhibit cancer	
	May enhance immune system	

From Shari Lieberman and Nancy Bruning, *The Real Vitamin and Mineral Book*, 2nd ed. (Garden City Park, NY: Avery Publishing Group, Inc., 1997). Reprinted by permission.

CARBOHYDRATES

Carbohydrates are needed to fuel the body and create energy. Complex carbohydrates are found in whole grains, beans, nuts, fruits, and vegetables. The body digests these complex molecular structures slowly, which makes these foods more filling than simple sugars, which are digested quickly and cause a rapid rise and fall of blood sugar levels. In addition, such starchy foods are generally relatively high in vitamins and minerals. They also contain more fiber than simple sugars and refined carbohydrates such as white bread; fiber aids digestion, prevents constipation and hemorrhoids, and helps prevent colon cancer and possibly breast cancer. Fiber also lowers cholesterol and blood sugar and thus also may protect you from heart disease and diabetes.

PROTEIN

We need protein to repair and replace cells and because it is the building block for biochemicals such as enzymes and brain chemicals. But be aware that eating too much protein contributes to a host of health problems, including heart disease, colon cancer, osteoporosis, and constipation.

FAT

Your body needs fat to carry certain "fat-soluble" vitamins, such as A, D, E, and K, through the system and to absorb minerals. Fats are also a part of our cell membranes and are needed to produce hormones. As a nation, we consume far too much fat—the equivalent of six to eight tablespoons daily. All we really need is the equivalent of about one tablespoon of high-quality fats per day; this can be obtained from a whole-foods diet with the addition of small amounts of high-quality cooking oils, salad dressings made with appropriate oils, and fresh nuts.

Saturated fat tends to raise cholesterol and is implicated in cardiovascular disease. Recent studies link breast and ovarian cancer to a diet high in saturated fats. Animal products are the main source of saturated fats, but some vegetable oils, such as palm and coconut oil, also contain saturated fat. You can tell when something is saturated fat because it remains solid at room temperature. Hydrogenated vegetable oils have been chemically changed into saturated fats by adding hydrogen atoms; they are used in margarine and processed foods such as pastries and baked goods to increase shelf life.

Polyunsaturated fats appear to lower cholesterol in the blood and may be less promoting of heart disease than are saturated fats; however, both saturated and unsaturated fats are implicated in many types of cancer, including colon, breast, and uterine cancer, partly due to this fat's vulnerability to oxidation. In fact, heating polyunsaturated fats creates free radicals. Vegetable oils such as corn, sunflower, and sesame are high in polyunsaturated fats.

Monounsaturated fats seem to be beneficial in that they actually lower LDL (the bad cholesterol) while raising HDL cholesterol (the good kind). The oleic acid in olive oil appears to protect fats from oxidative damage from free radicals. In addition to olive oil, peanut oil contains monounsaturated fats, as do avocados and cashews.

Essential fatty acids (EFAs) are called essential because they are essential for health and because our bodies cannot manufacture them. EFAs have many remarkable qualities. They are used in forming and balancing a group of hormonelike substances called *prostaglandins,* which regulate inflammation. They are found in every cell of our bodies and make the membranes more permeable. An imbalance of EFAs has been linked with increased susceptibility to infections and other immunological disorders such as allergies and arthritis, hair loss, mood swings, dry skin, cancer, cardiovascular disease, and reproductive problems.

Beware of Antinutrients

The term "antinutrients" sometimes is used to describe substances that work against good nutrition, in some cases by depleting the body of health-building nutrients. Some antinutrients, such as protein and saturated fat, are health-building nutrients but are harmful when eaten in excessive amounts. Others, such as caffeine, alcohol, and tobacco, are harmful in themselves. They are addictive substances that we use in excess to make us feel good temporarily. They are a drag on all the systems of your body and make your immune system work extra hard, leaving too little power to combat colds and flu. It's a challenge to kick the antinutrient habit, but it's well worth it because of the payback you'll get in better health and long-term well-being. Here's how.

CUT DOWN ON CAFFEINE

Caffeine is clearly America's favorite drug. It's found in coffee, black and green tea, cola drinks, chocolate, and many prescription and nonprescription medications. We like it because it perks us up and helps us think more clearly and quickly. The down side is that, in some people, caffeine causes "coffee nerves," anxiety, heart palpitations, sleep disturbances, gastrointestinal problems, urinary tract inflammation, and breast tenderness. Because it acts as a diuretic, it pushes your kidneys into overdrive and depletes your body of many nutrients including vitamin C, B-complex, calcium, magnesium, and zinc. Switch to decaffeinated beverages, herbal teas, cereal beverages, or plain hot water.

CUT DOWN ON ALCOHOL

With its relaxing effect alcohol acts as a "social lubricant" and enhances our enjoyment of food. Used in moderation, it appears to raise the level of "good" cholesterol in the blood (HDL). Studies done with men indicate that moderate drinkers live longer than teetotalers. But alcohol also has many negative effects, especially if consumed in excess. Alcohol depletes many B vitamins and minerals from the body and contributes to osteoporosis. It interferes with the way our bodies utilize vitamins and metabolize carbohydrates. It can wreak havoc with our efforts to eat a healthier diet, since it weakens our resolve to stay away from junk food, increases our appetite, or may cause us to forget to eat at all! Excess alcohol damages the liver, reducing its ability to metabolize toxic substances; it can be toxic to your heart and nervous system. Alcohol has been linked with an increased risk of breast cancer and other cancers. Alcohol has been shown to trigger hot flashes, accelerate aging of the skin, worsen premenstrual syndrome, and cause depression and sleep disturbances.

If you use alcohol at all, limit yourself to 4 ounces wine, 10 ounces beer, or 1 ounce hard liquor once or twice a week. Substitute light or nonalcoholic beverages such as wine coolers, ''near beer,'' iced tea drinks, and spritzers made with wine or fruit juice.

CUT DOWN ON FAT

The standard American diet gets 40 percent of its calories from fat—much of it saturated fat. Cutting down on fat would not only help you lose weight, it would help reduce your risk of cardiovascular disease, osteoporosis, many cancers, diabetes, stroke, and high blood pressure. The simplest way to cut down on fat is to emphasize whole, fresh, unprocessed foods such as vegetables, fruit, and whole grains. You'll get an added bonus of more vitamins, minerals, starch, and fiber; many studies suggest that it's the combination of low fat and high micronutrients that lowers risk of serious disease the most.

Avoid adding unhealthy fat—such as margarine and mayonnaise—to foods and cook using a minimum of fat. If you do use oil, make it olive oil (especially healthful for cooking) or cold-pressed polyunsaturated oil such as canola.

CUT DOWN ON PROTEIN

Most of the protein we consume comes from animal products, such as beef, chicken, turkey, pork, fish, eggs, milk, and cheese. Because protein is so concentrated in animal products, cutting your intake of these foods is by far the best way to bring your protein down to a healthier level. Replacing some animal proteins with vegetable proteins—beans, legumes, grains, nuts, and seeds—is wise, too, because vegetable sources can contain more vitamins, minerals, carbohydrates, and fiber and come "packaged" without the saturated fat found in animal products. You'd be wise to keep your protein down to about 15 percent of your total calories; think of it more as a condiment than as the star attraction of a meal.

CUT DOWN ON SUGAR

Sugar is a highly refined carbohydrate, and Americans eat an average of 150 pounds of sugar and other sweeteners every year. Our collective sweet tooth is a health problem for many reasons. Refined sugar contains only calories and no nutrients; if your body doesn't spend them as energy, they turn into fat. In addition, as your body uses sugar to create energy or as the excess is converted to be stored as fat, it depletes its own stores of nutrients, including B vitamins and the minerals chromium, zinc, and copper. High sugar intake also increases the excretion of nutrients such as calcium, magnesium, and chromium; in addition, sugar limits our ability to absorb calcium.

To cut down on sugar, emphasize fresh fruit instead of baked goods and candy. It's best not to try to appease or tease a sweet tooth, but if you have an overwhelming craving, try carrots or carrot juice—although high in sugar, they are also rich in fiber and antioxidants and can be easily taken "on the road."

CUT DOWN ON SALT

Salt, or sodium chloride, is a mineral needed to maintain water balance in our cells. However, modern Americans consume far more than the 2,000 milligrams (mg) needed each day: from 12 to 36 times more than we need! Most of the sodium sneaks into our diet from processed foods rather than the salt shaker. A serving of canned soup contains 1,500 mg sodium. Too much sodium contributes to high blood pressure in many people. Because it encourages your body to retain too much water, it may aggravate premenstrual symptoms such as bloating, headaches, breast tenderness, and irritability. Excess sodium causes calcium to be excreted in the urine, contributing to osteoporosis.

Presumably because salt was scarce during most of human existence on earth, we evolved a sodium-conserving mechanism. Today salt is no longer so precious, but we still conserve sodium in our bodies—and as our kidneys age and slow down, we conserve even more. To cut down on sodium, eat fewer processed foods and read labels carefully. Reduce the salt you use in cooking and seasoning; gradually substitute herbs, spices, powdered garlic, and lemon juice.

Immune-Enhancing Herbs and Spices

Certain herbs, spices, and flavorings are a delicious way to improve the immune power of your diet as well as perk up the flavor. It pays to keep the following culinary items on hand and incorporate them into your favorite recipes.

GARLIC

As long ago as ancient Greece, Rome, China, and Egypt, garlic was noted for its ability to stave off infection. Garlic eaters appeared to be able to resist the plague better, and during World Wars I and II, garlic helped troops recover from typhus, dysentery, and battle wounds. We now know something about why garlic—and other members of the lily family such as onions and leeks—has such power. Garlic contains many immune-supportive ingredients, such as vitamins B and C and selenium; it contains sulfur-containing compounds that act against bacteria, viruses, fungi, and parasites; it also lowers cholesterol and protects against cancer. Ten cloves of garlic have been found by some to be as effective an antibiotic as the average dose of penicillin. In fact, at one time it was known as Russian penicillin. As always, however, consult your health care practitioner before altering any prescribed medications. Although garlic capsules and deodorized garlic products are available, some experts believe that the best way to get the beneficial effects of garlic is to eat it, and raw is best of all. The usual recommended dose is at least 1 to 3 medium cloves per day, but if you really like garlic, there's no harm in eating more, except perhaps to your social life!

Since cooking may destroy the principal active ingredient, allicin, one way to retain the immune-enhancing effect while making it more palatable is to pickle the garlic cloves. In a screw-top jar, mix together ¼ cup each apple-cider vinegar, honey, and soy sauce. Add peeled garlic cloves, as many as will fit in the jar and still be fully immersed in the pickling solution, and place in your refrigerator for two weeks, until pickled. This will keep, refrigerated, for one month or more.

As a way to overcome garlic breath, you can eat raw parsley after a garlicky meal.

GINGER

Ginger is a proven antinausea herb, but studies show it also can boost immunity. Along with another aromatic spicy kitchen staple, garlic, ginger lowers blood pressure and cholesterol and reduces incidence of blood clots. You can use fresh grated, sliced, or diced ginger in your cooking; it's a welcome addition to any stir-fry recipe. Aim to include 1/3 to 1 ounce in your diet daily, especially during the cold and flu season. As a change from your usual beverage, try the Ginger Tea (page 89), as a preventive as well as a cold and flu remedy.

MAGIC MUSHROOMS?

Scientists are becoming increasingly interested in the medicinal properties of certain mushrooms. The most interesting mushrooms have been used in Asia for thousands of years and have immune-enhancing and antiviral effects. These include shiitake and maitake, two delicious, edible species. Their primary immune-active ingredients appear to be polysaccharides—large, complex molecules of carbohydrates. Shiitake is the most popular mushroom in Japan and is now available in the U.S., in either fresh or dried forms at health food stores, farmers' markets, and Asian markets. Recent studies using the extract of this mushroom have shown antitumor, antiviral, and immune-stimulating effects as well as other benefits, such as lower cholesterol and lower blood pressure. Studies with maitake concentrates and extractions have shown a profound effect on cancer, and there are anecdotal reports on people with chronic fatigue and HIV. Experts believe we can extrapolate these effects on the immune function and assume these mushrooms also would increase resistance to colds and flu and help your body handle an infection once it takes hold.

Reishi, a woody, bitter mushroom, can be made into a tea but is more palatable to Western tastes when taken in capsule form. Reishi also affects immunity: It appears to increase the activity of T-cells and macrophages, and have antitumor activity in animals.

So explore the produce department of your supermarket or health food store, farmers' market, or Asian markets if you have any near you and add an ounce or two of these mushrooms to your next soup, stew, or stir-fry, or eat the Immune Tonic Soup (recipe on page 83) once a week as a preventive.

Food as Cold and Flu Therapy

When you're sick—feverish, coughing, achy—most likely the last thing on your mind is food. This is the body's wisdom speaking up loud and clear. Most experts advise that it's best to eat sparingly and emphasize fluids during an illness in order to lighten the load on your system and preserve energy to battle the infection. However, choosing wisely the food you *do* eat can influence the speed with which you recuperate from an illness.

The foods suggested in the following pages have been tested for hundreds of years in kitchens and sickrooms all over the world. They are "comfort" foods, such as soups and stews, that soothe the body as well as the soul; antiviral foods such as hot teas; and immune-enhancing foods, such as garlic and other spices. Food may be the simplest and least expensive of cold and flu remedies. It certainly can be the most delicious. In choosing the healing foods for you, let your taste be your guide. If the thought or taste of a food feels right, then your body probably is telling you that you need it. If it doesn't taste appealing, then feed your body and soul with something else.

Comfort Foods Plus: Hot and Liquid

All warm or hot beverages and foods are helpful because they loosen phlegm and liquefy mucus, while bringing soothing warmth to ravaged tissues. If you include garlic, ginger, and medicinal mushrooms as ingredients, they also can boost immunity.

CHICKEN SOUP

Moses Maimonedes, a doctor-philosopher of the twelfth century, recommended it. Today the Mayo Clinic and Mount Sinai Medical Center both have endorsed the healing powers of this humble dish, also known as Jewish penicillin. Even these high-powered scientific institutions can't pinpoint the exact magic ingredient. (And perhaps they never will, if, as grandmas have alleged, it is their love.) But controlled laboratory studies show that chicken soup is a more potent cold remedy than plain hot water. One theory is that chicken is a food high in protein and therefore contains an amino acid called *cysteine.* This is coaxed out of the chicken and into the water when you make soup. Cysteine is very similar to a drug called *acetylcysteine,* which just happens to be used to treat bronchitis in respiratory infections because it thins out mucus and makes it easier for you to expel it.

So find a chicken soup recipe you like and keep it on hand for emergencies; if you can ask Grandma for the family recipe, so much the better. It helps, too, if you add spices such as pepper and ginger to the soup because they are expectorants that help rid viruses from your body. If you like the taste, add garlic ("Russian penicillin," see page 79) because of its antimicrobial and immune-enhancing ability; as they say, "it can't hurt."

CHICKENLESS CHICKEN SOUP

According to the work of a University of Nebraska researcher named Stephen Rennard, there must be more to chicken soup than chicken. Rennard tested his wife's grandmother's recipe and found that it reduced the inflammation-producing ability of certain white blood cells. However, this particular recipe, which included onions, sweet potatoes, carrots, turnips, and parsnips, was therapeutic even before the chicken was added. When he tested the five vegetables individually, each one appeared to have an anti-inflammatory effect. So it seems that almost any vegetable soup will help you feel better during a cold or flu.

MISO SOUP

For a therapeutic vegetarian soup, start with 1 quart vegetable stock (homemade, canned, or from boullion cubes). Add at least 4 cloves garlic and simmer until the garlic is just tender. Blend, and then add at least 1 tablespoon miso (soybean paste). Not only is miso fermented and delicious, but it will help your digestive system stay balanced if you are taking antibiotics for a bacterial infection.

IMMUNE TONIC SOUP

Make your favorite homemade soup, adding several slices of astragalus (see Chapter 7) root and a handful of fresh or dried shiitake or maitake mushrooms (see page 80). Simmer, covered, for 1 hour. You can eat the mushrooms, but remove the astragalus before eating. Eat one bowl per day during an infection, or one bowl per week for prevention.

KICHAREE

Kicharee is a medicinal meal that was used traditionally in Ayurveda (Indian medicine) to bring very sick people back to health. This vegetarian stew makes for a delicious, restorative meal whenever you are recovering from an illness. There are many different recipes for kicharee, so feel free to substitute other vegetables for those specified in this version.

   1/4 cup split mung dahl (yellow lentils, available at
      Indian food stores)
   1/2 cup basmati rice
   2 T. ghee (clarified butter) or sunflower oil
   1/4 tsp. cumin seeds
   3 bay leaves
   1 tsp. coriander
   1 tsp. oregano
   1/2 tsp. turmeric
   4 to 6 cups water
   salt to taste
   1 stick kombu (a type of seaweed)
   1 tsp. grated fresh ginger root
   3 cups diced fresh vegetables such as carrots,
      zucchini, and summer squash

Wash the beans and rice until the water runs clear. Warm the ghee or oil in a medium saucepan; add the cumin, bay, coriander, and oregano. Brown slightly until their aroma is released. Stir in turmeric, rice, and dahl. Add water, salt, kombu, and ginger. Simmer, covered, over medium heat for about ½ hour, or until beans and rice are soft. Add vegetables and cook 10 to 15 minutes, or until tender.

A Spot of Tea

The British and the Japanese, in their cold and chilly climates and homes that often lack central heating, may be on to something. Both countries are known for their bottomless teacups. It turns out that tea—both black and green tea—contains substances called *polyphenols*. Recently researchers tested tea extracts containing polyphenols and discovered that they inhibit the activity of both influenza A and B viruses when exposed to dog cells in test tubes. In comparison, amantadine, an antiviral drug, needed to be 50 to 100 times more concentrated than the polyphenols to get the same effect. Black and green teas also contain tannins, which are antioxidants. So, in addition to the soothing qualities of sipping a flavorful hot beverage, ordinary tea may have medicinal qualities. And if you feel the need for the lift that caffeine provides, consider tea instead of coffee.

Drink C and See?

Many people swear that drinking copious quantities of orange juice or other high-vitamin-C fruit juices make their colds or flu go away faster. One old family cold cure involves drinking, for each of one or two days, an entire can of pineapple juice diluted with an equal amount of water. However, there's no evidence that the vitamin C content in food is responsible for any perceived therapeutic effect. Although a recent study showed that 2,000 mg vitamin C can reduce the severity of a cold, this amount would be difficult to get just from food and usually requires supplementation.

Still, it's smart to eat or drink foods rich in vitamin C during a cold or flu. For one thing, drinking fluids—any fluids—is a wise strategy. Fruits are light and easy to digest, and many encourage urination, which may help detoxify your body. For another thing, even if you are taking vitamin C supplements, there may be substances in the food that enhance the absorption or utilization of the vitamin in pills.

Orange juice is the traditional high-C fruit elixir, but don't forget other fresh fruits high in vitamin C and other health-building nutrients, such as strawberries and other berries, grapefruit, pineapple, papayas, cantaloupe, and mangos. Any combination of these fresh fruits thrown in a blender makes a delicious smoothie that may soothe a dry, scratchy throat. Another favorite way to get your vitamin C is a hot toddy made with the juice of half a lemon and honey to taste.

A potent, edible source of vitamin C is amla or amalaki, the fruit of the Indian gooseberry. One berry is about the size of a plum and contains the same amount of vitamin C as seven oranges. You may be able to find this exotic fruit in a specialty produce shop if you live in a big city that has an Indian population. Otherwise, you may take 1 to 2 teaspoons powdered amla two to three times a day. It is available by mail from The Ayurvedic Institute, PO Box 23445, Albuquerque, NM 87192, 505-291-9698.

Note: Do not eat or drink citrus fruits or any food high in vitamin C along with zinc lozenges because citric acid deactivates the zinc.

GOT MILK?

Many natural health practitioners believe that drinking milk and eating dairy products such as cheese and ice cream stimulate your body to produce excess mucus and increase the risk as well as the severity of colds, flu, sinusitis, and ear infections. They say that this is an added burden on your respiratory, digestive, and immune system, and when you've got a cold, who needs that? Though adopting a dairy-free diet is controversial even among alternative practitioners, there is some evidence that milk contains a substance that stimulates the production of histamine, which turns on the runny-nose faucet.

Your Kitchen Pharmacy

The medicinal herbs you'll be learning about in Chapter 7 will likely mean a special trip to the health food or herb store. If a cold or flu strikes suddenly, why not try some of the many herbs and spices that you probably have on hand in your kitchen right now? Culinary herbs and spices are not only delicious; they also can be mild, safe, and natural medicines. The immune-enhancing herbs, garlic and ginger, and mushrooms recommended in the section on prevention also can be helpful during an illness. You can use them to add flavor to your favorite healing recipes or as directed below.

GARLIC OIL

Garlic oil is useful in easing symptoms of cold, flu, and fever. To prepare the oil, place 8 ounces peeled, minced garlic in a glass jar; cover with olive oil. Close tightly and set in a warm place for three days, shaking it three times every day to distribute the garlic. Press to extract as much of the garlic juice as possible, then strain the oil through a clean cotton cloth. Store in a cool place. Oil of garlic, along with cayenne pepper capsules, is an excellent remedy to take with you when you travel. Take 1 teaspoon garlic oil every hour to every four hours (depending on severity of symptoms).

GARLIC SYRUP

This palatable concoction is used to ease coughs, colds, sore throats, and bronchitis. To prepare the syrup, place 1 pound peeled, minced garlic in a two-quart glass jar. Add 2 cups each apple cider vinegar and distilled water. Cover tightly and place the jar in a warm place. Shake three times a day for four days. Then add 1 cup glycerin, available at pharmacies; let stand one more day. Strain the liquid through a cotton cloth, pressing the garlic into the cloth to extract as much of the juice as possible. Finally, stir in 1 cup honey. Store in a cool place. Take 1 tablespoon syrup of garlic three times a day before meals.

ONION-HONEY SYRUP

This is an old-fashioned cough remedy. Place 1 finely chopped raw onion in a small saucepan and add enough honey to cover. Cover, and cook over low heat for about 40 minutes. This syrup is reportedly so tasty that even children like it. Besides being antimicrobial, onions contain substances that help you expectorate mucus. They also create warmth, increasing the blood flow to your chest and throat. Take 1 teaspoon every 15 to 30 minutes, until symptoms subside.

GINGER TEA

Ginger aids digestion and is reputed to help cleanse the body by promoting perspiration, and fresh ginger teas are favorite herbal remedies for colds, flu, and fever. Ginger also contains a bronchodilator (useful in asthma) and reduces inflammation. One method to make ginger tea is to take a piece of fresh ginger root the size of a checker. Peel away the tough outer skin and cut into smaller pieces. Put 6 ounces water in a blender and start it whirring; then drop in the ginger until blended. Pour the mixture into a saucepan and bring to a boil; add 1 teaspoon honey to sweeten, if desired; you also may add 1 clove peeled, crushed garlic, 1 tablespoon fresh lemon juice, and 1/4 teaspoon cayenne pepper. Drink as much ginger tea as you want throughout the day.

BASIL TEA

For fever, make a tea of 1 ounce dried basil leaves and 2 cups water; you may add 6 peppercorns. Simmer for 20 minutes; strain, and drink as often as needed.

BLACK PEPPER

Black pepper is traditionally used in Indian medicine to help warm the body, which enhances immune response. Honey is an expectorant used to help expel the virus from the body. Mix together 1/8 teaspoon of black pepper (freshly ground, if possible) with enough honey to form a paste. Take three or four times a day for colds and sore throat. Another way to use black pepper is to brew a black pepper tea. Add 10 whole peppercorns to 1 cup water, cover, and simmer for 30 minutes. Remove the peppercorns, add honey, and drink while hot, up to four times a day.

CAYENNE PEPPER

For general cold and flu relief, take ¼ teaspoon powdered cayenne three times a day. To protect your digestive tract, you may put the powder in gelatin capsules (available in health food stores and pharmacies) and take 2 capsules every four hours. Or you may take cayenne powder in food as a daily tonic to prevent illness. Another use for cayenne is as a gargle; the pepper depletes the pain-causing chemicals produced by nerve endings and this relieves pain temporarily. Mix at least ⅛ teaspoon cayenne with ½ cup warm water, 1 tablespoon salt, and 2 tablespoons lemon juice. Gargle for as long as you can, but do not swallow.

CORIANDER TEA

To relieve fever, make a tea of 2 teaspoons crushed coriander seed in 1 cup boiling water; let steep 20 minutes. You may add a pinch of black pepper to increase the potency. Take three times a day until the fever lessens.

FENNEL TEA

To help expel mucus, drink a tea made of 1 teaspoon crushed fennel seeds in 1 cup boiling water; let steep 20 minutes.

ROSEMARY TEA

This aromatic herb makes a soothing tea during a cold. Simply add 1 teaspoon fresh rosemary leaves to 1 cup boiling water and let steep. Strain, and drink as needed to calm fever and an inflamed respiratory tract.

THYME SYRUP

Like ginger, thyme is used for high fevers; it also helps you expectorate mucus and is an antiseptic. To make a thyme-based cough syrup, add 1 ounce dried thyme to 2 cups boiling water; let steep for 10 minutes; strain and add 1 cup honey for sweetening if you wish. Take 1 teaspoon every hour.

THYME TEA

This is a favorite soother for sore throats. Pour 2 cups boiling water over 2 teaspoons dried thyme leaves; let steep, covered, for 15 minutes. Strain and sweeten with a little honey if desired; drink three times a day. You can even use this tea for a soothing gargle.

EUCALYPTUS AND SAGE INHALER

Use this herb combination to ease congestion and relieve a cough. In a saucepan, place 1 quart water and about 3 tablespoons each eucalyptus and sage leaves. Simmer for five minutes; remove from heat and let steep, covered, for 5 minutes. Remove the lid and place your head over the steam, using a towel to make a tent to capture the steam. Inhale for up to 15 minutes several times a day. For essential oils that you can use the same way, see Chapter 7.

Other Considerations

You also may want to consider other practices and possibilities, particularly if you are prone to frequent colds and flu. You may have allergies or sensitivities that are taxing your immune system, leaving you more vulnerable to infection. Or you may want to consider switching to organic food to reduce the toxic burden on all your systems. Finally, periodic fasting is a practice that may give your immune system just the boost it needs.

CHAPTER SIX

Vitamin and
Mineral Supplements

Eating according to the guidelines in the previous chapter will go a long way toward keeping your immune system in shape. But science has progressed beyond doggedly insisting that you can get everything you need from food. You may not even get enough vitamins and minerals to prevent obvious deficiency diseases such as scurvy. With few exceptions it's impossible to get the higher amounts that new studies show bestow optimum health and have therapeutic effects. So, along with eating a good diet, taking supplements is part of a comprehensive cold and flu prevention and treatment program.

In this chapter you'll find out how to get the most out of supplements. First you'll read why supplementation is becoming increasingly accepted and recommended. Then you'll learn which specific nutrients, and in what amounts, have been found to be beneficial during an established cold or flu. This is followed by a section on how to use supplements for optimal health, immune enhancement, and cold and flu prevention. And finally this chapter provides a primer on how to buy, store, and take supplements as well as what precautions to take.

Why Take Supplements?

While a nutritious diet is still the mainstay of good health, many studies and surveys have shown that the standard American diet leaves much to be desired. It's a rare bird indeed who obtains the Food and Drug Administration's Recommended Daily Allowances (RDAs) for all the vitamins and minerals. The RDAs were established by the National Academy of Sciences to provide a safety margin for essential nutrients that would prevent deficiency diseases such as scurvy, pellagra, and beriberi. (In 1993 the RDAs were replaced by the RDIs—Reference Daily Intakes, which represent the *average* need; they are essentially the same as the RDAs.) That's why it's wise to take a daily vitamin-mineral formula that supplies at least the RDA for all the known vitamins and minerals.

But recent studies show that the RDAs may not be enough for optimum health. Although the RDAs were a significant step in improving nutrition in this country, many respected authorities no longer believe they are adequate for every person. The RDAs often fall far short of creating and maintaining optimum health; nor are they adequate if you have health problems and are trying to recover your health. Many exciting new studies show that higher amounts of certain nutrients, such as beta-carotene, vitamin E, and vitamin C, enhance immune function, protect the respiratory system, and have many other beneficial effects as well. So many people report that they feel better when taking supplements in potencies higher than the RDAs that it's clear that some people need these higher amounts. Therefore, you may want to take so-called therapeutic doses of certain supplements in order to both treat and prevent colds, flu, and many other illnesses. What follows is a summary of the reasons that many natural health advocates believe most—if not all—of us should be taking supplements to ensure good health.

It Takes Planning to Eat a Balanced Diet

A large survey showed that less than 10 percent of the population eats the recommended minimum of five servings of fruits and vegetables daily, which makes the RDAs beyond their reach. Numerous other surveys have confirmed that Americans as a group are not getting even this minimum amount from their diet. It's easy to understand why. Even if we know what's good for us, we convince ourselves that our lives are too busy and unpredictable, and that good food isn't always available, so we settle for a quick toaster pop-up for breakfast, pizza for lunch, and burgers for dinner. In addition, a diet that satisfies the RDAs of vitamins and minerals is based on 2,000 calories—too high for most women to maintain their weight, even if they are active.

Nutrient Tables Are Unreliable

Foods vary tremendously in their nutrient content. Oranges are touted as a good source of vitamin C, but the vitamin C content of your orange juice may not be as high as the food charts say. Nutrient content varies depending on the growing conditions, how the crop was fertilized, and when it was harvested. Shipping, storing, and preparing all reduce the nutrient content of foods. For example, in the fall, a freshly harvested potato has 30 milligrams of vitamin C, but this drops down to 8 milligrams by spring and to zero in summer. English studies found that some Brussels sprouts have 64 times the chromium of others, and some wheat had 36 times more than other types of wheat. In addition, organic foods have higher levels of nutrients and fewer pesticides that can tax your immune system—factors ignored in nutrient tables. This means that "official" numbers may not be exactly what you are getting; in reality, you may be getting far less.

Individual Requirements Vary

We all are born with our individual biological blueprints, which include nutrient requirements and predisposition to diseases. In addition, we are under an unprecedented amount of physical stress from our polluted environment and psychological stress from our complicated, hectic lives. While such stresses are known to deplete the body of nutrients, we have evidence that supplemental nutrients help protect us against damage from such stresses. Furthermore, diseases and disorders—and many medical treatments themselves, even antacids, fiber supplements, and birth control pills—affect nutrient absorption and requirements, as does aging.

Scientific Evidence Is Building

There is plenty of evidence—and it is increasing every day—that taking supplements not only helps improve immunity and strengthen your respiratory tract but also can increase energy and mental alertness and reduce risk of major diseases such as cancer and heart disease. For example, two prestigious publications, the *Journal of the American Medical Association* and the *University of California at Berkeley Wellness Letter,* recently recommended that all Americans should take at least some nutritional supplements.

What to Take When You're Sick

Studies show that two major nutrients—one vitamin and one mineral—have an effect on an already established cold or flu: vitamin C and zinc. Studies also suggest that supplements are most effective and safest when you take the full spectrum of vitamins and minerals, not just one or two. Thus, if you decide to take C or zinc, be sure to take a full-spectrum multivitamin-mineral formula as well.

Vitamin C

You might think that the "C" in vitamin C stands for "controversy"—for that has been the history of this vitamin beginning in 1970, when the late Nobel Prize laureate Dr. Linus Pauling began singing its praises. Ever since his book *Vitamin C and the Common Cold* was published, this essential nutrient has been the subject of study after study, some of which have documented the benefits of supplementation, some of which have not.

Recently a researcher at the University of Helsinki in Finland analyzed 21 studies of vitamin C and colds. He found that vitamin C supplements may not be able to prevent a cold or flu but that when taken in large amounts, they can ease symptoms and shorten a cold's duration. Elliot Dick, the cold researcher at the University of Wisconsin who studies how colds are transmitted (see Chapter 1), also has studied vitamin C and the cold. He incorporated supplements of 2,000 milligrams (mg) a day (in divided doses) in one of his experiments. The students who took the vitamin C did not experience a significant reduction in the number of colds they caught, but they did have significantly milder symptoms. Over 20 other studies show similar results.

How does vitamin C reduce symptoms and hasten a

cold's departure? Vitamin C is a proven anti-inflammatory, evidenced by its value in treating allergies and asthma—and remember, inflammation contributes to cold and flu symptoms. And several studies suggest that vitamin C affects various white blood cells: It stimulates the production of lymphocytes; is required by the thymus gland, which produces T-cells; increases the effects of phagocytes, which "eat" bacteria, viral cells, and cancer cells; increases levels of interferon; and softens the effects of a stress hormone, cortisol, which dampens immunity. In many laboratory (test-tube) studies, vitamin C has inactivated a variety of viruses and bacteria. Other studies show that vitamin C is needed to maintain collagen, the protein that gives skin, tendon, bone, cartilage, and connective tissue their structure—remember, a strong respiratory tract is your first defense against cold and flu viruses and bacteria. One study suggested that vitamin C can prevent chronic bronchitis.

So, how much vitamin C should you take when you're sick? Studies show you need to take at least 2,000 mg (2 grams) per day—and some studies used doses as high as 6,000 milligrams. In this range, cold symptoms and duration were reduced by about 30 percent. Doses under 1,000 mg were ineffective, and nutritionists have observed that patients who take less than this do not relieve symptoms or shorten the duration of colds. Thus, many nutritionists advise taking 2,000 mg a day during a cold or flu, and still others suggest you take 3,000, 4,000, or more . . . up to 10 or 15 grams. They say that when you are sick, your body can absorb and utilize much more vitamin C than when you are well and that your body will let you know how much you need through a phenomenon called "bowel tolerance." The first time you take large doses of vitamin C while sick, they recommend you start with

1,000 or 2,000 mg a day, and add 1,000 mg each day until you notice symptoms of gas, bloating, or diarrhea. Then cut back down on the dosage so that bowel symptoms disappear. Linus Pauling recommended taking 1,000 mg every hour that you are awake, which adds up to 16,000 mg, whether you are sick or not!

How you take vitamin C is as important as how much you take. The doses should be divided over the course of the day. For example, if you are taking 3,000 mg, take 1,000 mg with each meal. After your cold or flu symptoms have abated, be sure to taper off gradually, so your body has a chance to adjust. Some practitioners recommend you use the powdered ascorbate form because it is more easily absorbed. Other than bowel symptoms, there are no confirmed adverse effects to taking large doses of vitamin C; earlier studies that suggested kidney stones might occur have been disproved.

Zinc

Many studies show that zinc boosts immunity, but only recently have health professionals been recommending zinc supplements to reduce symptoms during a cold. We owe this new twist to a little girl who, in 1978, accidentally performed an experiment on herself. The girl, who was being treated for leukemia, decided to suck on her zinc tablets, which she was taking to counteract the immune-depleting effects of the chemotherapy. Lo and behold, the cold she had disappeared. Her father persuaded researchers to investigate, and sure enough, allowing zinc tablets to dissolve slowly in the mouth and throat seemed to work as a cold remedy. Swallowing zinc supplements without allowing prolonged contact with the throat does not have the same effect.

An important study of patients in the Cleveland Clinic supports this use and helped refine the treatment. The 1996 study reported that in patients who took zinc lozenges, cold symptoms disappeared 42 percent faster than patients who took placebos (sugar pills). Symptoms lasted approximately four days compared with eight days, and symptoms of sore throat, coughing, and nasal congestion were particularly affected. However, the patients taking zinc also suffered some unpleasant side effects: They had 30 percent more nausea than those on the placebos and 50 percent more bad taste in the mouth. So, in considering zinc lozenges, you need to balance these risks against the possible benefits. The researchers admit that no one knows for certain why zinc reduces symptoms. But there are several theories: Zinc seems to inhibit the virus from reproducing; it may prevent the virus from entering the cell; it appears to step up production of interferon; and it also may reduce inflammation.

How much to take? In the Cleveland Clinic study each lozenge contained 13.3 mg zinc gluconate. Patients were instructed to take one lozenge (or placebo) every two hours while awake for a total of seven or eight lozenges a day, for the duration of their colds (up to 18 days). In reality, they took an average of four to eight a day, but as the researchers point out, this lower dose seems to have been effective.

Zinc gluconate by itself tastes awful and takes a long time to dissolve. Specially formulated lozenges made of zinc gluconate taste better than ordinary zinc supplement tablets and dissolve better too. Still, some people object to the taste, so you might try sucking on a honey lozenge along with the zinc. Also, the nausea that some people report can be lessened if you take the lozenges after a meal. Aside from nausea, there are no known side effects if you take even large amounts of zinc for a short period of time; in the above-mentioned study, the average daily dose adds up to 53.2 to 106.4 mg. However, some nutritionists advise that you not exceed 50 to 60 mg a day for the duration of treatment. Zinc is most effective when begun within 24 hours after symptom onset.

Supplements for Prevention

Supplements can be helpful before you get sick too. Scientific evidence is growing that certain supplements can boost immunity and strengthen the respiratory tract, thus giving us added protection against colds, flu, and many other diseases and conditions. Although few studies involve colds and flu specifically, many involve the immune system and diseases (such as cancer) that are related to immune function.

Most of the positive studies using supplements (rather than food) involve the antioxidant nutrients that protect our respiratory tract tissues and immune systems from free radical damage. (Free radicals and antioxidants are discussed on pages 61–62 in Chapter 5.) Studies do suggest that doses in excess of the RDA for the antioxidant nutrients vitamins E, C, and A and beta-carotene and the minerals zinc and selenium are particularly useful in enhancing immunity and reducing the risk of infection (and the other diseases and conditions associated with free radical damage). There's even some evidence that supplements can reverse these diseases or help slow their progression once they are established.

However, since nutrients work together in the body, and there may be as-yet undiscovered synergistic affects, the best strategy for boosting immune function is to take all the antioxidants along with the full spectrum of other vitamins and minerals. Refer to the table at the end of this chapter for the Recommended Daily Allowances, the Optimum Allowances, and the safety limits on vitamin and mineral supplementation.

VITAMIN C

As discussed earlier, vitamin C has many beneficial effects on the immune system, and levels of vitamin C in white cells drop when we have colds or other infections. Studies have shown that vitamin C supplements enhance immunity in elderly people. Although no studies have shown that vitamin C supplementation can prevent colds, many people have noticed this effect, and studies do show that it can prevent colds from being severe and from lingering.

ZINC

Zinc, also discussed on pages 98–100, is required in adequate amounts for proper immune functioning. This mineral is depleted when upper respiratory infections are accompanied by fever. Studies in which elderly people were given 220-microgram supplements daily showed improvement in their immune systems.

VITAMIN A AND BETA-CAROTENE

Vitamin A and its precursor, beta-carotene, have been shown to enhance immunity in both animal and human studies. Vitamin A lowers the rate of infections of the respiratory system, and beta-carotene in high doses may increase the levels of T-cells. A recent study demonstrated that 50 mg beta-carotene every other day improved the level of natural killer cell activity in elderly men, which may improve their resistance to viruses and cancer. Beta-carotene also may protect your respiratory system from smoke and air pollution, allowing it to withstand viral invasion better. Many human population studies associate diets high in vitamin A and beta-carotene with lower incidence of many forms of cancer, including lung cancer.

Clearly, large amounts of beta-carotene can be beneficial, but the case for supplementation is not so clear-cut. Recent studies raise disturbing questions about the effectiveness and safety of supplementation when beta-carotene is taken alone. Over 600 carotenoids have been identified, but only a few of them have been found in human blood and tissues; these include alpha-carotene, beta-carotene, lutein, zeaxanthin, cryptoxanthin, and lycopene. Research suggests that other carotenoids may be as effective or more effective than beta-carotene and that the carotenoids are more powerful when they act together. Unfortunately, mixed carotenoid supplements are much more expensive than beta-carotene alone. And unlike many other nutrients, it is possible to get high amounts of beta-carotene from diet alone, and in food they are accompanied by the other beneficial carotenes. Some people, therefore, prefer to rely on food—orange and yellow fruits and vegetables such as winter squash, carrots, and cantaloupe—and others eat these foods but also take beta-carotene supplements.

VITAMIN E

This vitamin has been shown to enhance almost every aspect of the immune system—resistance to infection, antibody response, and the activity of lymphocytes and phagocytes. Other studies suggest that vitamin E is needed to maintain healthy macrophages, T-cells, and B-cells. Studies on elderly people have shown that 800 IU of vitamin E supplement daily can enhance immune response, supporting earlier work that indicated that high levels of vitamin E in the blood lower the incidence of infection among the elderly.

SELENIUM

This mineral activates glutathione peroxidase, an antioxidant enzyme produced by the body. Studies show that selenium supplementation activates phagocytes and is anti-inflammatory. Selenium is known as an anticancer mineral because so many studies equate high intakes or blood levels with a lower rate of many types of cancer.

The National Cancer Institute is conducting ongoing "chemopreventive" trials of several individual nutrients including selenium, vitamin E, and vitamin A. However, these nutrients tend to work synergistically. For example, when large doses of selenium and vitamin E were given together to experimental animals, antibody production increased up to 30 times; and vitamin C is needed to prevent vitamin E itself from doing free radical damage.

OTHER NUTRIENTS

Other supplements containing substances that are not quite vitamins or minerals also may help build immunity and repel colds and flu. Three of the most studied have been discussed in Chapter 5: flavonoids, a group of antioxidants that help fight viral infections; garlic, an antioxidant, antiviral, and immune enhancer; and omega-3, an essential fatty acid and immune enhancer. These are included in the chart "Nutrient Table of Vitamins and Minerals" on pages 106–07.

Other supplements are less well studied, including Pycnogenol, the name of a patented blend of flavonoids extracted from the bark of the European coastal pine tree. Pycnogenol appears to be a very powerful antioxidant—in test tube studies, it was 20 times more powerful than vitamin C and 50 times more effective than vitamin E. You may wish to add this to your prevention regimen, particularly during the flu season. The recommended dose is 100 to 150 mg for two to four weeks, tapering off to 50 mg per day.

How to Begin Your Prevention Program

The ''Nutrient Table of Vitamins and Minerals'' on pages 106–07 gives a range of safe, recommended dosages for the best-known nutrients. Take these amounts year-round for general good health; you may wish to increase the dosage of vitamin C during the cold and flu season. The chart shows you both the RDA and the Optimum Intake.

The Optimum Intake amounts are based on the most current research studies published in professional journals and the experiences of well-respected clinicians. More is not always better where nutrition is concerned. The range of optimum amounts recommended may seem high to those who follow the RDAs, but these dosages are beneficial for many people. If you have any questions or concerns, work with a nutritionist or physician knowledgeable in nutritional sciences.

Since vitamins and minerals typically work together, look for a multiple vitamin-mineral formula as your foundation. Then add individual supplements such as vitamin C to achieve the total desired dosages, where appropriate.

How to Buy and Take Nutritional Supplements

Keep the following in mind when buying and using supplements:

• For increased effectiveness, try to divide the dosage throughout the day. For example, if you are taking 1,500 mg vitamin C, take 500 mg three times a day.

• Take most supplements with meals; doing so increases absorption and prevents indigestion or "tasting" the vitamins later. Amino acid supplements should be taken on an empty stomach; iron supplements should be taken separate from calcium because these two nutrients compete for absorption in the digestive system.

• Some experts believe that you should buy only "natural" vitamins because synthetic ones are less effective. Others feel that you are paying extra money for nothing. Keep in mind that the accepted definition of a "natural" nutrient is one that has a chemical structure the same as that found in nature. We can synthesize such chemicals easily, yet they are labeled "natural" because it is believed the body can't tell the difference. However, some natural products are more biocompatible than synthetic vitamins—that is, they are more easily absorbed and therefore better used by the body. For example, there is evidence that this is true of the naturally occurring form of vitamin E. There is also evidence that food concentrates that are naturally high in certain nutrients are also better absorbed and utilized. However, in most cases, high potencies are difficult to get in natural form.

• Store supplements in a cool, dark, dry place—not the refrigerator, which is damp. Supplements have a limited shelf life, so toss them after the expiration date.

NUTRIENT TABLE OF VITAMINS AND MINERALS

Nutrient	RDA/ RDI*	Optimum Intake†	Safe Intake‡	Possible Toxicity
Vitamin A	5,000 IU	5,000–20,000 IU	10,000 IU	21,600 IU
Beta-carotene	none	40,000–100,000 IU	43,332 IU (25 mg)	
Vitamin B complex		25–300 mg each		
B-1	1.5 mg		50 mg	
B-2	1.7 mg		200 mg	
B-3	20 mg		500 mg	1,000 mg
B-6	2 mg		200 mg	500 mg
Vitamin B-12	6 mcg	25–500 mcg	3,000 mcg	
Folic acid	400 mcg	400–1,200 mcg	1,000 mcg	5,000+ mcg
Pantothenic acid	10 mg	25–500 mg	1,000 mg	
Biotin	300 mcg	300 mcg	2,500 mcg	
Vitamin C	60 mg	500–5,000 mg	1,000 mg+	
Vitamin D	400 IU	400–800 IU	800 IU	2,000 IU
Vitamin E	30 IU	400–1,200 IU	1,200 IU	
Vitamin K	80 mcg	80 mcg	30 mcg	
Calcium	1,000 mg	1,000–1,200 mg	1,500 mg	2,500 mg+
Magnesium	400 mg	500–600 mg	700 mg	uncertain
Iron	18 mg	15–30 mg	65 mg	100 mg

Nutrient	RDA/ RDI*	Optimum Intake†	Safe Intake‡	Possible Toxicity
Selenium	70 mcg	50–400 mcg	200 mcg	910 mcg
Zinc	15 mg	22.5–50 mg	30 mg	60 mg
Copper	2 mg	2 mg	9 mg	uncertain
Omega-3	none	250–3,000 mg	none	
Garlic	none	200–1,200 mg	none	
Flavonoids	none	250–1,000 mg	none	

Important Precaution: If you have any diagnosed health problem or special health needs, consult a physician on the proper and safe nutrient dosage for you.

* RDA values are for nonpregnant, nonlactating adults.
† Partially adapted from Shari Lieberman and Nancy Bruning, *The Real Vitamin and Mineral Book,* 2nd ed. (Garden City Park, NY: Avery Publishing Group, Inc., 1997). Reprinted by permission.
‡ Safety levels based on *Vitamin and Mineral Safety,* prepared by the Council for Responsible Nutrition, Washington, D.C., 1997. Used with permission. "Safe intake" is the level at which there are no credibly-substantiated adverse reactions observed in humans; however, you should consult your health care practitioner about appropriate levels for you.

"Possible toxicity" is the lowest intake at which some adverse effects have occurred under certain circumstances. For many nutrients, to date there are no reports of any adverse effects at any level and thus these entries have been left blank.

Precautions

As a general rule, it's best not to take a supplement of just one nutrient. Nutrients typically work synergistically and frequently depend on one another to work best. For example, you need adequate amounts of calcium and magnesium plus other minerals and vitamin D to slow osteoporosis. In addition, taking large doses of one nutrient can create an imbalance in your body. If you take only vitamin B-12, for example, it competes with other B vitamins to be absorbed in your intestine, and an excess of B-12 could create a deficiency in the others. The B vitamins usually work best together.

Remember, nutritional supplements are just that—*supplements* to a healthful, balanced diet and active lifestyle, not *substitutes*. Taking supplements is not a license to slather margarine over everything, lie around eating junk food, or smoke cigarettes.

If you have a diagnosed disease and/or are taking medication, consult a professional before taking supplements. Some supplements may interact with medication or cause problems. The recommended dosages have been found to be safe in the vast majority of people; however, be alert for any possible side effects or unusual sensitivities.

CHAPTER SEVEN

Herbal Medicine

Herbs have come a long way—or have they just come full circle? Today you don't need to go to a health food store or health food restaurant to find herbs and herbal teas. Now even pharmacies and supermarkets stock teas, pills, and tinctures, and you usually can find at least a few herbal teas on the menu of most restaurants, fast food emporiums, and coffeehouses. Herbal teas are a healthy alternative to caffeinated coffees, black teas, and sticky-sweet sodas—but they are much more, too. Herbs can be potent medicines and play a significant role in both treating and preventing colds and flu.

According to Rob McCaleb, president of the Herb Research Foundation, over 1,800 herbs are sold in the United States today. Americans spent an estimated $1.6 billion in 1996 on herbs. Although "herbs" refers to the above-ground parts of plants, herbalists use this term to include all plants as well as mushroom remedies that might be more accurately referred to as "botanical substances."

This chapter is a basic primer on how herbs work and

how to buy, prepare, and use them medicinally. You'll find descriptions of the most commonly used herbs and herbal formulas used to enhance immunity and relieve specific symptoms as well as "tonic" herbs to strengthen your immune system and help prevent colds and flu from taking hold. You'll also learn about aromatherapy and how to use fragrant herbal oils to soothe symptoms. Remember, although many herbs are generally safe for most people, just because they are "natural" doesn't mean they never have any detrimental side effects. Before taking any herb medicinally, check with your medical practitioner, particularly if you are pregnant, nursing, or have a diagnosed medical condition. And be sure to read the general precautions provided on pages 139–42 of this chapter.

How Herbs Work

Herbs are called "nature's pharmacy" and have been used for thousands of years to treat just about every disease and condition you can think of. Although they work in a similar way to conventional drugs—by their biochemical effect—herbal remedies are generally gentler and safer.

Few people realize that many of the drugs used in conventional medicine are derived from herbs. For example, digitalis is made from foxglove and aspirin originally was made from the white willow. Some herbal agents were tested long ago, and fascinating accounts of these studies exist in old medical texts. But even many physicians don't realize that although much of our knowledge of herbs comes from folk medicine, herbs also have been studied scientifically and more and more articles are being published in prestigious medical journals.

And herbs are being tested by manufacturers and naturopathic doctors, especially in other countries. In Germany, for example, herbalism has evolved into phytotherapy (plant therapy). That country has set up a special agency devoted to evaluating herbs using the same methods and standards used to evaluate drugs. In the United States, however, virtually all herbs are in regulatory limbo—they are not officially approved by the Food and Drug Administration (FDA) because the agency considers them to be foods, not drugs.

So, welcome to the increasingly scientific world of herbs. In this chapter you'll find herbs such as echinacea, astragalus, and goldenseal that relieve your symptoms and increase resistance to disease by boosting your immune system. Others, such as elecampane and licorice, promote expectoration of mucus and ease coughs due to colds. Still others, such as boneset, ginger, and elder flowers, are diaphoretics that encourage perspiration and thus help break a fever and eliminate the virus through the skin.

What all these various herbs and mechanisms of action share is the underlying principle that plants contain constituents which work together synergistically. In contrast to conventional medicine, rather than isolating a single "active agent," herbal therapy uses the whole plant or whole parts of the plant such as leaves, flowers, or roots. Doing so can increase their effectiveness while decreasing the side effects that may occur when using isolated components.

How to Buy and Use Herbs

You can buy single herbs and herbal formulas in various forms at health food stores, food co-ops, herb stores, and farmers' markets, as well as from health practitioners and mail-order companies. Most busy people prefer the convenience of commercially prepared herbs in tincture, extract, or pill form (tablets or capsules). But herbs are also available in loose form, and you can use these for making your own teas, decoctions, and infusions and even your own tinctures, extracts, and capsules if you wish. Don't overlook the added advantage of taking your herbs as hot teas, infusions, or decoctions—drinking warm liquids has a therapeutic effect all its own where colds and flu are concerned.

Because the FDA doesn't regulate the contents of herbal products, there's no guarantee of the herb's purity or how much active ingredient is in a particular plant or bottle. Freeze-dried or tincture forms from reputable companies are usually the most effective and consistently potent. See Appendix A for a list of herb suppliers with a reputation for high-quality products.

BUYING LOOSE HERBS

When buying loose dried plants, look for a bright color and a strong flavor and aroma; organic herbs are preferable. Two to four ounces of each dried herb is a good amount to start with and keep on hand. Store them in a tightly closed container, such as a small glass jar, and keep them in a dark dry place (not the bathroom medicine cabinet, which can be too damp and hot) for up to one year. (Mark the expiration date on the container.)

What Form to Take?

Although prepackaged herbal teas are widely available, they may not be potent enough to be considered medicinal. The following forms, listed in increasing order of potency, are considered to best extract and activate the medicinal properties of herbs.

HERBAL TEAS

Teas are brewed for a short time and are an easy and pleasant way to take herbs. To make tea, pour boiling water over the loose herbs or tea bag. Generally, about 1 to 2 teaspoons loose herb per cup of water is recommended; or you may use 1 ounce of herb per 2 cups water. Let steep for 5 to 10 minutes; remove the herbs from the water before drinking. (Longer steeping results in a bitter brew.) Teas are the least concentrated form and are useful mostly for mild symptoms. For medicinal purposes, you may make a more medicinal cup of tea by tripling or quadrupling the usual amount of herbs (three to four tea bags) and steeping for a full 10 minutes; this is more equivalent to the more potent decoctions or infusions described next. Cover the pot or cup when steeping, as volatile oils such as in peppermint may evaporate before you drink them.

Begin cautiously and drink only half a cup the first time. If you experience no adverse reaction, you can gradually increase the amount you drink. Generally, one cup equals one dose.

DECOCTIONS

Decoctions are made by boiling the herb. Break up the hard, woody parts of plants—stems, roots, and bark—into small pieces so there is a greater surface area from which the healing chemicals can be released more readily into the water. Add 1 ounce herb to 3 cups water; boil for about 10 minutes until the water is reduced down to 2 cups. Next add the rest of the plant—leaves and flowers—

and cover and steep for another 10 minutes. Strain the mixture and store in your refrigerator for up to 3 or 4 days. Generally, the dose is one to three cups per day. (Note: If you are using a combination of herbs to prepare a decoction, use 1 ounce total combined herbs, not 1 ounce of each herb.)

INFUSIONS

Infusions are made by pouring boiling water over the dried flowers or leaves of the herb. Be sure to break them up or crush them first in a clean cloth. Use 1 ounce herb and 3 cups boiling water. Cover and let steep for 20 to 30 minutes. Strain and refrigerate for up to 3 or 4 days. One to two cups per day is the usual dose. (Note: If you are using a combination of herbs to prepare an infusion, use 1 ounce total combined herbs, not 1 ounce of each herb.)

TINCTURES

Tinctures are concentrated preparations of herbs that have been preserved in alcohol. Most people get their tinctures from an herbalist or herb company. Alcohol-based tinctures last almost indefinitely if stored in a cool, dark place; some are made with cider vinegar, which remains potent for about one year, or glycerin, which may have a longer shelf life. You take tinctures by the drop— about 10 to 30 drops three times a day—or by the tea-spoon—about 1 per day. Taking the tincture as drops straight from the bottle dropper under your tongue will get them into your system the fastest, but the alcohol makes the herbs unpleasant to take this way. Most people prefer to add the tincture to a small amount of boiled water to make a beverage—the hot water evaporates the alcohol.

EXTRACTS

Extracts are also highly concentrated preparations of herbs, but unlike tinctures, they are prepared with water. However, they usually have glycerin or alcohol added as preservatives. They are taken in the same manner as tinctures.

CAPSULES OR TABLETS

Pills contain dried herbs and are the most convenient form for busy people. They are less likely to turn moldy than are loose herbs, and they also retain potency for about one year. Some herbalists dislike capsules and pills because they feel the active constituents are not as readily available to your body in this form. There's no guarantee that your digestive system will release the healing agents to the same degree as the heat, water, and alcohol used in preparing the other forms. Dosage varies widely but is generally 2 capsules or tablets two or three times a day. Follow the directions on the bottle unless advised otherwise by an experienced doctor or herbalist.

CHINESE HERBS

Chinese herbs usually are formulas that the practitioner combines specifically for each individual patient; the loose herbs and other natural substances are boiled to make a strong tea. Patent remedies for colds and flu are available without a prescription in health food stores and Chinese pharmacies.

Seeing a Professional Herbalist

Most people are able to use herbs to take care of themselves during a cold or flu and to improve their overall health and resistance by using tonic herbs. However, if you find you still get frequent colds or flu, and the symptoms linger or turn into bronchitis or sinusitis, you may have a deep-seated immune problem that is best treated professionally. An herbalist will be able to guide you in using herbs to treat the acute illness and its symptoms and to treat the underlying condition that led to the infection. During a visit with an herbalist, expect to be evaluated physically, emotionally, and mentally. As a natural health practitioner, the herbalist will spend whatever time is needed to determine the imbalance and disharmony that is at the root of your condition.

Unfortunately, there is no certification or licensing process in this country specifically for herbalists. However, many licensed medical doctors (M.D.'s), nurse practitioners (L.N.P.'s) naturopathic physicians (N.D.'s), and acupuncturists use herbal medicine. To find one of these health professionals who is licensed to practice in your state, ask for referrals from friends who are under the care of an herbalist, or inquire about local herbalists at your health food store. You also may contact the organizations in Appendix A for referral to a knowledgeable herbalist in your area.

Once you have one or more names, call their office and ask where they studied herbalism and how long they have been practicing it. The School of Medical Herbalism and its affiliates have an excellent reputation for producing well-trained herbalists. You also may ask the herbalist for the names of clients you can call for reference.

Using Single Herbs for Colds and Flu

What follows is an alphabetical glossary of the individual herbs most commonly used to treat colds and flu. You'll find particular emphasis on echinacea and goldenseal since these are the two "stars"—the immune-boosting herbs most often prescribed for common infections. Follow the suggested dosages for these and the other herbs unless directed otherwise—either by the labeling on an herbal product or your practitioner. Dosages assume the person taking the herbs weighs about 150 pounds; for smaller or larger individuals, adjust the dosage accordingly. Herbs generally are best taken along with meals.

These same herbs are often used in combination; using single herbs helps you determine which specific ones work best for you and reduces the chance of an adverse reaction. If you don't notice any improvement, try another herb or combination formula. If that doesn't work, then move on to the next.

Aniseed

This licorice-flavored herb has been used since ancient Egyptian times and makes a delicious tea that traditionally is used to soothe coughs and colds.

Use in Colds and Flu: Coughs.

Preparation and Dosage: Steep 1 teaspoon crushed aniseeds in 1 cup boiling water. Drink 2 to 3 cups a day.

Astragalus

This ancient Chinese herbal remedy traditionally is used to increase resistance to disease. Studies from China have demonstrated that astragalus may both lower the incidence of colds as well as shorten their duration. A potent immune system strengthener that enhances interferon production, it generally is used as a preventive tonic for general disease resistance and increased energy. It also may be used at the first sign of a cold or flu to shorten the duration and lessen the severity of the symptoms.

Use in Colds and Flu: Strengthens the immune system.

Preparation and Dosage: The generally recommended daily dosage is:

1 (300–400 mg) capsule, up to 3 times daily; or
1 teaspoon tincture, up to 3 times daily; or
15 to 30 drops extract, up to 4 times daily (check dosage on label).

Balm of Gilead

Balm of gilead, taken from tall poplar trees, is mentioned several times in the Bible. It soothes the body's mucous membranes lining the respiratory tract.

Use in Colds and Flu: Sore throat, cough, bronchitis, and laryngitis.

Preparation and Dosage: The generally recommended dosage is:

Syrup: 1 tablespoon, up to 3 times a day.
Tincture: 2 teaspoons up to 3 times a day.

Bayberry

This is a spicy herb that traditionally has been used during the early stages of a cold, flu, or cough. It is said to improve the immune response and encourage perspiration for fever reduction.

Use in Colds and Flu: Cough and Fever.

Preparation and Dosage: To each 1 cup boiling water, add 1 teaspoon bayberry bark; let steep, covered, until it has cooled down to a drinkable temperature. Add honey if you wish, and drink as needed to ease symptoms. You also may gargle with the tea to soothe a sore throat.

Boneset

Also known as feverwort, boneset is a traditional Native American herbal remedy used to treat fevers, colds, and flu. It is a diaphoretic herb, meaning it promotes perspiration, which in turn helps break a fever. Boneset eases the aches and pains that usually accompany flu and sometimes accompany colds.

Use in Colds and Flu: Fever and flu.

Preparation and Dosage: The generally recommended dosage is:

   4 to 10 capsules, up to 3 times daily; or
   1 cup infusion, up to 3 times daily; or
   10 to 40 drops extract daily.

Cayenne

Also known as capsicum, cayenne is a common herb and traditionally is used to help you sweat out symptoms of colds, flu, and bronchitis. It is also rich in vitamin C and antioxidants.

Use in Colds and Flu: General symptom relief, bronchitis, cough.

Preparation and Dosage: The generally recommended dosage is:

   1 capsule, up to 3 times daily; or
   1 cup tea daily; or
   1 teaspoon tincture, up to 3 times daily; or
   1 tablespoon syrup (the most common form), up to 3 times daily.
   1 teaspoon tincture, up to 3 times daily.

Precautions: Capsicum should not be used if you have hemorrhoids, hyperacidity, or gastrointestinal ulcer.

Chaparral

Also known as creosote, chaparral is known as an antibiotic, antiviral herb. It is used for cold and flu and any inflammation of the respiratory system.

Use in Colds and Flu: General symptom relief.

Preparation and Dosage: The usual dosage is:

1 cup infusion, 3 times daily; or
10 to 30 drops tincture, 3 times daily.

Precautions: There are potentially dangerous side effects if this herb is used incorrectly. Therefore, many practitioners recommend that you use this herb only under the guidance of an experienced professional. Pregnant and nursing women should not use chaparral, nor should people with lymph or kidney problems.

Cleavers

Also known as clivers or goose grass, cleavers has many traditional uses. For colds and flu, it is favored for its ability to restore an inflamed, swollen lymphatic system, an important component of the immune system, and for cooling down fevers.

Use in Colds and Flu: Fever.

Preparation and Dosage: The generally recommended daily dosage is:

5 to 10 capsules, up to 3 times daily; or
½ to 1 teaspoon tincture, up to 3 times daily; or
1 cup infusion, up to 3 times daily; or
½ to 1 teaspoon extract, up to 4 times daily.

Damiana

Damiana traditionally is used as an aphrodisiac and also is an effective treatment for mucus congestion and the coughs that arise from this consequence of colds and flu.

Use in Colds and Flu: Cough and congestion.

Preparation and Dosage:

1 cup infusion, 3 times daily; or
10 to 30 drops tincture.

Echinacea

Of all the dozens of herbs used to treat colds and flu, echinacea is the queen. Also known as the purple cone flower, echinacea (eh-kih-NAY-sha) has a long history of use in this country, but until recently has been popular primarily in Europe. Native Americans used echinacea centuries ago for a huge variety of ailments and injuries, and, starting in the 1870s, doctors in the U.S. prescribed it for coughs, colds, and sore throats. This flowering herb fell out of favor when antibiotics became available in the 1930s. But, according to a report in *Chemical and Engineering News* in the fall of 1996, echinacea is now the top-selling herbal medicine in the United States. It has been reported on by the *Wall Street Journal* and *USA Today*—a sure sign of recognition by the mainstream. Echinacea has been studied extensively, particularly in Europe. In addition, researchers at Bastyr University Research Institute (a naturopathic college in Seattle) and Dalhousie Medical School in Nova Scotia are launching separate studies of the herb in an attempt to replicate some of the European research.

Echinacea contains a diverse array of active components that affect different aspects of immune function.

Echinacea reportedly raises levels of white blood cells when they are low. In animal experiments, the herb seems to have positive effects on the immune system by increasing white blood cells and phagocytes, which engulf and destroy bacteria and other pathogens.

Laboratory studies suggest that echinacea extract fights bacteria and viruses including those associated with influenza. In addition, studies show that echinacea has polysaccharides that bind to the receptors on the surface of white blood cells and literally turn them on. Studies have shown that echinacea stops the formation of hyaluronidase, an enzyme that destroys the body's natural defense barrier against pathogens.

Many people swear that taking echinacea at the first sign of a sore throat or a cold or the achiness of the flu helps them avoid illness altogether—or, failing that, at least eases the symptoms and makes them go away sooner. In a 1992 study performed in Germany, people who took freshly pressed echinacea juice recovered from cold and flulike symptoms about two days faster than those who took a placebo (dummy preparation).

Echinacea comes in capsule form as well as tincture, but many herbalists prefer the tincture because, in their clinical experience, it seems to work better. You can drip the tincture directly on your tongue or mix it in water or juice. (You will notice that echinacea causes your tongue to tingle for a few minutes after taking it as tincture, decoction, and extract. This is not dangerous—it is a sign that the preparation is potent.) Many experts recommend in particular the fresh-pressed juice of the species of echinacea known as *purpurea* because it provides the greatest range of active compounds and has been used in the most impressive studies. Some health professionals prefer the brand Echinaguard, the product that was used in Germany in several positive clinical trials.

Use in Colds and Flu: Immune-strengthening and general symptom relief.

Preparation and Dosage: Frequency of dosage depends on severity of symptoms; for severe symptoms, you may take echinacea every 2 hours and gradually decrease the frequency to 3 times a day as symptoms improve. The generally recommended dosage is:

1 teaspoon (1 dropperful) tincture; or
1 cup decoction; or
15 to 30 drops extract; or
1 (300 mg) capsule.

Precautions: Echinacea shouldn't be taken during pregnancy or by people with tuberculosis or diseases thought to have an autoimmune component, such as lupus and multiple sclerosis. Some herbalists also warn people who are HIV-positive to use caution when using echinacea, especially over long periods, because the herb's effects in these people are unknown.

Elder

This herb is traced to the Gypsies, who use it for colds and flu; it is also useful for sinusitis. Elder often is used along with other herbs such as peppermint, ginger, or yarrow, in both homemade and commercial preparations.

Use in Colds and Flu: General symptom relief.

Preparation and Dosage: When used alone, the generally recommended daily dosage is:

5 capsules, up to 3 times daily; or
1 teaspoon tincture, up to 3 times daily; or

1 cup infusion, up to 3 times daily; or
½ to 1 teaspoon extract, up to 3 times daily.

Elecampane

Also known as horseheal, elecampane has been used in many cultures for centuries to treat many types of respiratory problems. It encourages expectoration and therefore is especially useful when you have a cough.

Use in Colds and Flu: Cough.

Preparation and Dosage: The generally recommended daily dosage is:

5 capsules, up to 2 times daily; or
1 to 2 teaspoons decoction, up to 2 times daily; or
¼ to ½ teaspoon tincture, up to 2 times daily.

Precautions: You should not use elecampane if you have diabetes.

Ephedra

This is an ancient remedy to reduce congestion of many upper respiratory conditions, with a history that goes back to ancient India. It is also known as *ma huang* in China, where it has been used to treat asthma. In fact, two components of ephedra are used to manufacture several nonprescription medications for asthma, bronchitis, and allergies. Because it stimulates the nervous system, ephedra is an ingredient in many weight-loss pills.

Use in Colds and Flu: Congestion, bronchitis.

Preparation and Dosage: The generally recommended daily dosage is:

5 to 10 capsules, up to 3 times daily; or
1 teaspoon tincture, up to 3 times daily; or
1 cup decoction, up to 3 times daily.

Precautions: Ephedra can cause insomnia, nervousness, and a dry mouth; it also may raise blood pressure and cause heart palpitations. Therefore, ephedra should not be used without professional guidance by anyone who is pregnant or nursing; has diabetes, a heart or thyroid condition, high blood pressure, or glaucoma; or is on any medication.

Eucalyptus

Also known as blue gum tree, eucalyptus is a native of Australia. Its leaves contain a powerful natural antiseptic, antibiotic, and expectorant, and are frequently used as a treatment for coughs, colds, flus, and other respiratory problems.

Use in Colds and Flu: Congestion.

Preparation and Dosage: Eucalyptus is the main ingredient in Vicks VapoRub, Tiger Balm, and other salves and liniments that mothers traditionally and lovingly rub on their children's chests to unclog breathing passages.

Precautions: Do not take eucalyptus oil internally.

Garlic

Garlic has a long history as medicine—this potent anti-infective was used as long ago as 3000 B.C. in ancient Sumeria.

Use in Colds and Flu: Immune and respiratory system strengthener.

Preparation and Dosage: You can use garlic as a medicinal food (see Chapter 5), as a nutritional supplement (see Chapter 6), or as seasoning in your favorite dishes. As a medicinal herb the usual dosage is:

½ to 1 teaspoon tincture, up to 4 times a day; or
2 to 6 capsules per day in divided doses.

Many of these capsules are deodorized or coated so you avoid that garlic smell. These products seem to be just as effective as the fresh, aromatic form.

Ginger

Ginger traditionally is used to calm nausea and improve digestion, but studies also show it stimulates the immune system and helps sweat out a fever. Many practitioners therefore recommend that during a cold or flu, you incorporate ginger into your regimen.

Use in Colds and Flu: Fever, antiviral.

Preparation and Dosage: Ginger is delicious and can be used as a medicinal food (see Chapter 5); as a medicinal herb, you may use the following dosages:

1 to 2 capsules, up to 3 times a day; or
1 teaspoon tincture, up to 3 times a day.

Precautions: Some people may find that ginger causes heartburn.

Goldenseal

Goldenseal, also known as yellow root, is known for its antibiotic and immune-stimulating abilities. Usually it is recommended for treating all types of respiratory problems including colds, flu, and bronchitis because it dries and cleanses the mucous membranes. Goldenseal is native to North America and was used extensively by Native Americans for many maladies of the respiratory and other systems. Many studies show that plants containing compounds called berberis alkaloids, such as goldenseal, are powerful antibiotics. (Other berberine-containing plants you might see on the market are Oregon grape, barberry, and goldenthread, which is used in China.) There is some evidence that goldenseal/berberis stimulates the immune system, particularly the macrophages that engulf and destroy viruses and bacteria. It may help reduce fever—not by suppressing prostaglandins, as is the case with aspirin, but by enhancing your immune system's ability to deal with substances that produce fever. However, some experts point out that goldenseal seems to be poorly absorbed by the body and thus may be useful only in treating infections along the gastrointestinal tract, not elsewhere in the body. They believe that you are on firmer ground with the herb echinacea, for which there is much better evidence of efficacy against colds and flu.

Goldenseal often is combined with echinacea in commercial formulas and used as a preventive as well as a treatment.

Use in Colds and Flu: Immune strengthening, antibacterial.

Preparation and Dosage: The generally recommended dosage is:

1 to 3 (300 mg) capsules, up to 3 times daily; or
$\frac{1}{2}$ to 1 teaspoon tincture, up to 3 times daily; or
1 cup infusion, up to 2 times daily.

Precautions: Goldenseal can raise blood pressure and thus should not be taken by anyone with high blood pressure.

Lemon Balm

This herb is a perspiration-inducing diaphoretic. It is particularly recommended for use in children because it tastes much better than most herbs and because it also has a calming effect. An ointment made with lemon balm has been shown to relieve herpes sores and thus may prove helpful for "cold sores."

Use in Colds and Flu: Fever.

Preparation and Dosage: For fever the usual dose is taken as a tea made of 1 ounce lemon balm leaves steeped in 2 cups boiling water, as often as needed.

Licorice

Licorice is a traditional remedy for coughs and inflammation and may help prevent infection. Often it is used in combination with other herbs.

Use in Colds and Flu: Coughs, lung congestion, and cold sores.

Preparation and Dosage:

1 capsule, up to 3 times a day; or
½ to 1 teaspoon tincture, up to 2 times a day; or
½ to 1 teaspoon extract, up to 3 times a day.

Precautions: Licorice may raise blood pressure and therefore should not be taken if you have a history of hypertension, diabetes, glaucoma, stroke, or heart disease; or if you are pregnant or nursing.

Linden Flowers

This herb, particularly when combined with chamomile, makes a delicious, soothing beverage during a cold or flu. As is the case with lemon balm, this diaphoretic tea is particularly appealing to children. A recent study conducted by two pediatricians at the University of Chicago found that children given linden blossom tea recovered more quickly from flu than those given any other treatment. Linden tea was ten times more effective than antibiotics and other drugs, which slowed recovery and caused more complications (middle ear infections).

Use in Colds and Flu: Fever, general symptoms.

Preparation and Dosage: The standard dose is:

> 1 ounce linden blossoms steeped in 2 cups boiling water for up to 20 minutes, taken as often as desired.

Myrrh

In tincture form, this herb helps ease pain and speed healing of cold sores. Apply several times a day, using a clean cotton swab each time.

Peppermint

This pleasant-tasting herb is a traditional remedy for colds, flu, and stomach upset. It is often part of a combination formula.

Use in Colds and Flu: Fever, general symptom relief.

Preparation and Dosage:

> 1 cup infusion made with 1 ounce herb and 3 cups boiling water; or
> 10 drops peppermint oil to 2 quarts water.

Red Clover Flowers

This herb also is called cow clover or purple clover. It is known for its immune-enhancing ability and for its antispasmodic and expectorant properties. Thus it often is recommended for coughs due to congested mucus.

Use in Colds and Flu: Coughs.

Preparation and Dosage: The usual dose is:

1 cup infusion, as needed; or
10 to 30 drops tincture, as needed.

Slippery Elm

This herb is a noteworthy emollient and was used traditionally by Native Americans as a soothing remedy for a variety of ailments. It also is an expectorant and thus helps soothe dry, irritated throats and quiet coughs.

Use in Colds and Flu: Coughs and sore throats.

Preparation and Dosage: Slippery elm is available as lozenges; or you may take it as follows:

1 teaspoon tincture, up to 3 times a day; or
1 to 3 teaspoons herb to 1 cup boiling water, for tea; let simmer for 15 minutes; up to 3 times a day; or
Mix the powdered bark with enough water and honey to form a thick paste. Take by the spoonful and let it dissolve slowly in your mouth, coating your throat with its soothing sweetness.

Tea Tree Oil

This remedy has become a popular item in health food stores and has been made into a huge variety of products for hair, skin, scalp, nails, teeth, and gums. The variety known as cajuput is useful for relieving congestion and coughs and for inducing perspiration during the early stages of colds and flu. You also may add tea tree oil to a vaporizer and inhale the aromatic steam, or apply directly to cold sores or canker sores.

Use in Colds and Flu: Sore throat.

Preparation and Dosage: The usual dosage for tea or gargle for sore throat is:

¼ to ½ teaspoon oil in warm water, up to 3 times a day.

Yarrow

Yarrow has a long history as a pain reliever and wound healer. When you have a cold, yarrow tea helps soothe canker sores.

Use in Colds and Flu: Canker sores.

Preparation and Dosage: Make a strong tea by steeping 3 teabags or 3 tsp. loose herb in a cup of boiled water; let cool and rinse your mouth as often as desired.

Precautions: Taken in very large amounts, yarrow can be poisonous.

Using Herbal Combinations

Individual herbs can be very effective and may be all you need. However, many herbalists recommend herbal combinations for their synergistic effects. You can buy commercially prepared formulas, or you may purchase herbs singly and combine them yourself, using the tried-and-true formulas that follow. Refer to the alphabetical listing of single herbs earlier in this chapter for background information and precautions for each herb.

In the following combinations, amounts refer to weight, not volume; for example, if 1 part equals 1 ounce, 2 parts equals 2 ounces. Dosages assume the person taking the herbs weighs about 150 pounds; for smaller or larger individuals, adjust the dosage accordingly.

Immune-Boosting Formula #1

Measure out 1 part each (⅕ ounce) echinacea root, goldenseal root, elder, peppermint, and yarrow, for a total of 1 ounce combined herbs. Begin by making a decoction of the echinacea and goldenseal roots; add the roots of these herbs to 3 cups water and boil for 10 minutes or until the liquid has been reduced to 2 cups. Add the remaining herbs and allow to steep, covered, for 10 minutes. Strain; drink up to 3 cups daily, until symptoms subside.

Immune-Boosting Formula #2

Here's another combination herbal formula designed to boost immunity during an infection. Since it needs to steep for several weeks, make it before the cold and flu season starts. Combine 2 parts ($^2/_5$ ounce) echinacea with $^1/_2$ part ($^1/_5$ ounce) goldenseal and 1 part ($^1/_5$ ounce) each finely chopped fresh garlic and grated fresh horseradish. Put the herbs in a quart jar, pour in enough vodka or brandy to cover them, plus 2 inches. Cover the jar and let the mixture steep for at least 4 weeks. Strain out the solids and pour into a smaller glass bottle. You may take 1 dropperful (about 1 teaspoon) 3 times a day, mixed with $^1/_2$ cup warm water.

Flu-fighting Formula

For flu, you may try the following combination of herbs: Combine 3 parts each ($^3/_{10}$ ounce) echinacea root, goldenseal root, and boneset with 1 part ($^1/_{10}$ ounce) peppermint, for a total of 1 ounce combined herbs. Boil the echinacea and goldenseal in 3 cups water until the liquid is reduced to 2 cups (about 10 minutes). Add boneset and peppermint and steep, covered, for another 10 minutes. Strain, and drink up to 3 cups daily.

Formula for Productive Coughs

For coughs that bring up phlegm or mucus (productive coughs), try the following combination, which acts as an expectorant to help bring up the mucus. Combine a total of 1 ounce elecampane root, ginger root, and licorice root (⅓ ounce each). Add the herbs to 3 cups water. Make a decoction by boiling for 10 minutes or until the liquid has been reduced to 2 cups. Strain, and drink up to 3 cups a day until your cough subsides.

Syrup for Dry Coughs

You can make an excellent cough syrup by combining equal parts of balm of gilead buds and elecampane with ½ part licorice; mix with enough honey to make a syrup. Take 1 tablespoon as often as needed.

Sore Throat Formula

Combine 1 part each elder, peppermint, and yarrow (⅓ ounce each) to total 1 ounce herbs. Add to 2 cups boiled hot water and let steep for 10 minutes. Strain, and drink up to 3 cups a day, until symptoms have subsided.

Bronchitis Formula

If your cold or flu develops into bronchitis accompanied by coughs that produce a lot of phlegm (productive coughs), try this combination. Combine equal parts (⅓ ounce) elecampane, goldenseal, and licorice, for a total of 1 ounce the combined herbs. Make a decoction by adding the herbs to 3 cups water and boiling for 10 minutes or until the liquid has been reduced to 2 cups. Strain, and drink up to three cups a day, until symptoms are eased. For bronchitis accompanied by a dry cough, use the Syrup for Dry Coughs.

Fever-Reducing Formula

Herbs don't try to eliminate your fever; they try to help your body use the fever in the most efficient way to help fight off infection and thus shorten its duration. A helpful herbal drink is made by combining 2 parts each ($^2/_5$ ounce) elder and yarrow along with 1 part ($^1/_5$ ounce) peppermint, for a total of 1 ounce combined herbs. Make an infusion of these herbs by adding them to 1 pint boiled water; cover and let steep for 10 minutes. Strain and drink up to 3 cups a day, until your fever breaks.

For greater convenience, you might try a new product called Fevera, from HerbaSway. Said to be effective in reducing fever as well as fever blisters, the herbal liquid concentrate is based on traditional Chinese medicine and contains standardized extracts of skullcap, Chinese kudzu, Chinese knotweed, licorice, and *Cassia tora*.

Chinese Herbal Formulas

Chinese herbs aim to balance the yin-yang (two forces) in the body that are out of kilter during an illness such as cold or flu. Chinese doctors prescribe many traditional recipes, and every Chinese household keeps them or variations of them on hand. In traditional Chinese medicine, the treatment varies from person to person, depending to a large extent on the person's constitution. You may buy commercially prepared formulas, in which herbs effective for colds and flu are already combined.

Two increasingly popular patented Chinese herb formulations are Gan Mao Ling and Yin Chiao San. They come in easy-to-take tablets and are sold in Chinese pharmacies and herb shops as well as health food stores. Gan Mao Ling generally is thought to be more appropriate for colds and contains herbs reputed to be antiviral and antibiotic. Many practitioners recommend this formula during a cold to ease symptoms and during the cold season as a preventive. Yin Chiao San contains herbs traditionally used to reduce inflammation and often is preferred for treating flu.

Preventing Colds and Flu with Tonic Herbs

Many herbs are known for their specific effects—they can soothe a cough, ease a fever, relieve a stuffy nose. Others have more far-reaching general effects—they nourish, support, and balance the body's systems, so they can function optimally. When herbs are used this way, they are said to "tonify," that is to say, they tone and strengthen your organs just as physical exercise tones and strengthens your muscles.

There's a long tradition, particularly in Chinese medicine, of taking tonic herbs. They are great for fostering overall health and providing extra insurance against a specific health problem to which you are at higher-than-average risk because of genetic predisposition or too much stress. Tonic herbs are particularly suitable for people who are "run-down," with low immunity and low energy. Tonics are used to establish and maintain a healthy condition and balance in order to prevent illness and to restore vitality after an illness. They are to be used as a complement to other health-building and restoring approaches such as diet, nutritional supplements, appropriate rest and activity, and stress management.

Generally, you take tonic herbs all year round or when you are under a lot of stress. They work slowly. It may take months to detect an improvement in your health and energy, so give a tonic two to six months before you decide whether it's helping or not. Tonifying herbs may be used singly or in combination. The most commonly recommended tonic herbs for boosting resistance against colds and flu are echinacea, astragalus, and ginseng.

Echinacea

Just as echinacea is the premier herb during an infection (see earlier discussion, page 121–23), so it is the premier immune-boosting tonic. A German study, using people prone to frequent respiratory infections, showed that those who took echinacea were less likely to get sick than those who took a placebo. Most herbalists recommend that you take this herb for eight weeks and then break for one week before resuming. Many people take it beginning a month or so before the cold and flu season, and then take it throughout the winter. Some herbalists recommend that you do not take the herb for more than about ten days in a row—not because it isn't safe, but because there is some evidence that echinacea seems to work better when taken in an on-off pattern and because the body may stop responding to the herb's immune-stimulating effects when it is taken continually. A study was published showing that when you take echinacea every day without a break, your phagocytes (the immune cells responsible for searching out and destroying viruses and cancer cells) rise to peak levels but do not stay there. They eventually drop back down to the baseline and stay there even though you're continuing to take the herb. Taking echinacea in a pulsed regimen ensures that your body continues to respond and your immune system remains enhanced.

Preparation and Dosage: The usual dose for echinacea as a tonic is:

> 1 capsule, up to 3 times a day; or
> 1 teaspoon tincture, up to 3 times a day; or
> 1 cup decoction, up to 3 times a day; or
> 15 to 30 drops extract mixed with water or juice, up to 4 times a day.

Precautions: As discussed, there is controversy over the duration of the use of echinacea for disease prevention.

Astragalus

In China, this tonic herb is used to boost energy, but in the West, it is used mainly as an immune-system strengthener. (See earlier discussion, page 117.) It is suitable for people who are overstimulated by ginseng (usually people under 40). You may take astragalus on a continual basis.

Preparation and Dosage: The usual dosage is:

1 capsule, up to 3 times a day; or
1 teaspoon tincture, up to 3 times a day.

American Ginseng (Panax quinquefolium)

American ginseng traditionally was used by Native Americans and is now used around the world. It is milder than Asian ginseng and is more appropriate for women who have not yet achieved menopause. Ginseng contains compounds called ginsenosides, which advocates believe are responsible for its overall tonic effects. It is known for helping people deal better with stress and fatigue and for its immune-stimulating properties.

Preparation and Dosage: The usual dosage is:

1 capsule, up to 3 times a day; or
1 cup decoction, up to 2 times daily; or
$1/2$ to 1 teaspoon tincture, up to 3 times a day.

Precautions: There have been reports of insomnia and allergic reactions that may have been due to use of American ginseng.

Panax Ginseng (Korean, Chinese, or Asian Ginseng)

Like American ginseng, this herb contains ginsenosides but is more powerful and stimulating. It has been used in Asia to boost energy, immunity, and sexuality, and to improve ability to handle stress. Ginseng has been shown to enhance antibody response, the production of interferon, natural killer cell activity, and the function of macrophages, phagocytes, and lymphocytes. It has been shown to prevent viral infections in animal tests. Asian ginseng is used primarily by men, since it contains testosterone; it is also suitable for postmenopausal women. Ginseng is traditionally used in an on-off pattern: two weeks on, two weeks off; it is generally recommended that you do not use ginseng during an illness.

Preparation and Dosage: The usual dosage is:

   1 capsule, up to 3 times a day; or
   1 cup decoction, up to 3 times a day; or
   5 to 10 grams powder in water or juice, in divided
      doses over the day.

Precautions: This herb may cause high blood pressure or irritability. Do not use Asian ginseng if you have high blood pressure, and avoid taking it close to bedtime if it causes sleeplessness. If ginseng makes you nervous or irritable, lower the dosage or discontinue use.

Immune-boosting Tonic Combination

You may want to try taking a combination of echinacea and red clover, which support your immune system, and yellow dock and dandelion root, which help eliminate toxins. The simplest way to take them is to buy the commercially prepared tinctures of all four herbs and combine them; take 1 teaspoon of this formula up to three times a day. Or make your own decoction, using equal parts of the loose herbs to total 1 ounce. Add the dandelion, echinacea, and yellow dock roots to 4 cups water, and boil for 10 minutes, until it has been reduced to 3 cups. Add the red clover flowers, cover, and let steep for another 10 minutes. Strain, and drink up to 3 cups daily.

General Precautions for Herbs

Be sure to buy herbs only from the most reputable sources you can find; several are listed in Appendix A. Quality and potency can vary depending on harvesting, handling, and storage; in addition, there have been reports of mislabeling of herbs. Because they are made according to certain standards, many practitioners recommend tinctures, freeze-dried products, and extracts as the safest and most effective forms of herbal remedies.

➤ Remember to use caution when self-prescribing herbs. Certain herbs may cause undesirable reactions in some people. Begin with the lowest recommended dosage of the purest form you can find, and increase gradually as needed. The most common symptoms of herb intolerance are nausea, vomiting, diarrhea, or allergic reactions; however, these are rare and extremely variable, depending on both the herb and the individual. Most side effects from herbs are idiosyncratic—they vary unpredictably from person to person. If you notice any questionable reaction, discontinue the herb(s) at once. If your reaction is severe, call your local Poison Control Center and go to the emergency room of the nearest hospital.

➤ Read the manufacturer's recommendations carefully, and make sure there is detailed information on appropriate dosages.

➤ If you are over 65, stick to the lowest dosage recommended.

➤ Although herbs are usually safe, do not combine them with prescription or over-the-counter medication unless you are under professional guidance; some herbs may contain substances similar to those in the medication and could result in an overdose. If you have any questions or doubts, contact a knowledgeable herb specialist for advice.

➤ Consult your health care practitioner before taking an herb if you have any medical conditions or if you develop any adverse side effects.

Aromatherapy

Aromatherapy uses aromatic herbs to help heal us on physical, emotional, mental, and spiritual levels. The Egyptians and other ancient peoples used fragrant oils, herbs, flowers, and other natural substances to treat and comfort one another. Today aromatherapy uses essential oils whose fragrance has the power to affect the part of the brain that regulates basic life processes and is also the seat of our emotions. It's no wonder that smells can so powerfully affect mood and well-being and help relieve symptoms of cold and flu.

How to Buy and Use Essential Oils

Essential oils are sold in tiny bottles or by the drop in health food stores, aroma shops, and food co-ops as well as through the mail. Some companies make combinations blended to relieve specific symptoms, such as headache. You need only a drop or two at a time, depending on the concentration of the oil—sometimes they are "cut" with a carrier oil. Well-sealed, fragrant oils have a long shelf life. Make sure you buy only pure and natural oils (not synthetic) made specifically for healing purposes.

FOR GENERAL RELIEF OF COLDS AND FLU

The most frequently used aromatic herbs to boost immunity are lavender, tea tree, and rosemary. For chest congestion, try eucalyptus, peppermint, camphor, and cedarwood. Tea tree, geranium, lemon, and black pepper are said to combat infection. For head colds and blocked sinuses, try basil, eucalyptus, and peppermint. For flu or heavy colds with fever, try camphor, eucalyptus, basil, black pepper, bergamot, chamomile, hyssop, melissa, or peppermint.

Fragrant steam: Perhaps the best way to use aromatic herbs during a cold or flu is to add them to a steam vaporizer or other source of steam, such as a bowl of hot water (see Chapter 4) and inhale them. This will help open up nasal passages, ease chest congestion, and clear blocked sinuses. For a more subtle effect, you also can add an essential oil to a steam vaporizer and let the steam heat diffuse the aroma throughout the entire room.

Fragrant bath: Another pleasant way to treat colds with aromatherapy is to soak in a hot bath to which you have added 3 drops lemon oil, 2 drops each thyme and tea tree oil, and 1 drop eucalyptus oil. Add the oil while the water is running into the tub, and soak for about 20 minutes. Be careful, since the oil is slippery.

Fragrant rub: Make your own soothing chest rub by combining 3 drops eucalyptus oil and 2 drops thyme oil to 2 teaspoons vegetable oil (such as sesame oil).

Massage as often as needed onto your chest and throat to open up clogged passageways. Or mix 3 drops sandalwood, 2 drops eucalyptus, and 1 drop peppermint oil with ½ fluid ounce carrier oil (such as sesame or almond oil). Apply the fragrant oil to your face, throat, and chest to ease a sore throat.

Fragrant hankie: Sprinkle 2 drops rosemary oil and 1 drop each geranium and eucalyptus oil on a clean tissue. Place under your nose and inhale to clear sinuses. Another traditional sinus opener is 2 drops eucalyptus and 1 drop each lavender and peppermint. DO NOT SWALLOW.

Precautions: Some people are allergic to certain essential oils. Take a sniff and test each one on a small spot on the back of your hand before purchasing or using on more delicate skin surfaces. Some oils may cause adverse effects in people with certain conditions, such as epilepsy or high blood pressure, so check with a knowledgeable professional if you have any of these problems. Do not take essential oils internally unless you are under a knowledgeable professional's care, since some can be harmful when ingested.

CHAPTER EIGHT

Homeopathy

Homeopathy often is confused with herbal therapy, but it is founded on completely different principles. Homeopathic remedies use substances not only from plants but also from the animal and mineral world. This gentle medicine developed as a reaction to the harsh methods of dealing with sickness in the eighteenth century, which included blood-letting and purging. Since its inception, homeopathy has been used to treat a wide variety of illnesses, including colds and flu. This natural medicine offers real help in terms of relieving symptoms of a current infection as well as strengthening the body's response to future infections. In fact, evidence suggests that homeopathy was more effective than conventional therapy during the great flu epidemics of the early 1900s. In this chapter you will learn about the most popular single and combination remedies used for colds and flu, and how to use them.

What Is Homeopathy?

Homeopathy is based on the principle that "like cures like," which grew out of the time-honored observation that substances that cause harmful symptoms in healthy people can, in very diluted doses, cure similar symptoms in sick people. So, for example, if you have a cold with runny nose and burning watery eyes, you may benefit from a homeopathic remedy called Allium cepa, which is made from onion.

Homeopathy was developed in the late 1700s by a German physician named Samuel Hahnemann. One day he was translating a scientific text about cinchona, a Peruvian bark that contains quinine. The text attributed cinchona's ability to alleviate the fever of malaria to its bitter and astringent properties. To Hahnemann, this made no sense, and he decided to test the substance on himself. After several doses, he noticed that he developed symptoms similar to those of malaria. Was this just coincidence, he wondered, or was this the mechanism behind the bark's effectiveness?

Hahnemann proceeded to test many other substances and discovered that the similarities were no coincidence. Eventually he began to treat patients by matching their symptoms with the medicines that had produced them in a healthy person. Amazingly, his theory was supported by his experience: The medicines worked! Like did cure like, and in this way, homeopathy was born. Hahnemann and his followers tested many more substances on healthy human subjects, always noting in careful detail the symptoms that the substances provoked.

By the way, the like-cures-like principle is not unknown in conventional medicine. For example, certain immunizing vaccinations use small doses of allergens; digitalis, which is toxic to the heart, is used in small doses for heart failure; small amounts of colchicine, which causes symptoms of gout, are used to treat this condition; and gold, which causes joint pain, is used to treat arthritis.

Homeopathy spread throughout Europe in the nineteenth century, partly based on its success in treating life-threatening infectious diseases. It has continued to have a loyal and substantial following in Europe—especially England, France, and Germany—and in India, Latin America, and the former Soviet Union. Homeopathy is the fastest-growing medicine in the world and is also growing in popularity in the United States.

Does Homeopathy Work?

Homeopaths point to historic evidence that the treatment is effective. They point out that homeopathy was far more effective than the prevailing conventional medicine during the terrible typhoid, cholera, and flu epidemics that swept through Europe and the United States in the 1800s. The death rates in homeopathic hospitals were as much as one-half to one-eighth the rate in orthodox hospitals. Homeopaths also present as evidence their own experience and their satisfied patients.

Experimental studies support the efficacy of homeopathy. In 1991 the *British Medical Journal* published an analysis of 107 clinical studies published between 1966 and 1990. The authors found that the homeopathic treatments were successful in 81 of the experiments. Even when they included only the 23 studies that they considered to be of the highest quality, the vast majority of these (15) showed positive results. The studies involved many conditions; interestingly, 13 out of the 19 trials of respiratory infection treatment were effective; six out of seven showed positive results for other infections. The authors of the analysis, who were nonhomeopathic Dutch physicians, said, "Based on this evidence, we would be ready to accept that homeopathy can be efficacious if only the mechanism of action were more plausible."

Two sets of studies have been conducted on two over-the-counter homeopathic remedies that also met with positive results. One group of studies tested oscillococcinum (ah-sil-oh-kok-SIGH-num), derived from duck heart and liver, of all things, for its ability to relieve flu symptoms. All three studies found it to be effective for fever, shivering, and symptoms due to flu. One of the studies, conducted in 1985, found that in the group who took the homeopathic product, fever decreased more rapidly—in two days—than in the placebo group; and shivering disappeared by day four. The second controlled study, published in 1989 in the *British Journal of Clinical Pharmacology,* found that 66 percent more of the oscillococcinum group recovered within 48 hours. Many animal and laboratory studies demonstrate homeopathy's ability to stimulate the immune system, inhibit the growth of viruses, and reduce opportunistic infections in people with HIV infection.

How Does Homeopathy Work?

Even homeopaths can't answer this question precisely. The remedies are prepared by a process called potentization that is used to make them safer and more effective. During this process, the original active substance is diluted, usually in a solution of distilled water or grain alcohol. The substance is diluted again and again—sometimes up to thousands of times. (See sidebar.) Most scientists are skeptical that something so diluted can have an effect.

In many remedies not even a single molecule of the original substance remains! However, as the above-mentioned studies demonstrate, homeopathy works very well in skeptical adults as well as young children and animals. You don't have to believe in it or understand the mechanism for it to work, and you have little to lose since homeopathic remedies are very low in cost and adverse effects are extremely unlikely in commonly used potencies. However, you may be curious to hear about the theory behind this unusual natural therapy.

The most common theory is that the shaking process used when the remedy is prepared or potentized "imprints" a memory of the remedy's energy pattern on the molecules of water or alcohol. This process retains the active substance's pure essence while preventing any harmful effects that the active molecules themselves may cause. For example, arsenic is normally a poison, but it is harmless when it is diluted homeopathically; however, it is a potent remedy for flu.

Homeopathy subscribes to the idea that symptoms are signs that your body is trying to deal with an underlying disorder or imbalance and therefore should not be suppressed. According to the principle of like cures like, taking a remedy that matches the symptoms of your illness stimulates and supports your symptoms and strengthens your body's innate healing power. Eventually your body no longer needs the symptoms and they fade away naturally.

Homeopathy recognizes that your symptoms are not just physical—they also can exist on an emotional and mental plane, and all three planes are interrelated. Homeopathic remedies, therefore, are prescribed according to your unique overall *pattern* of symptoms and general individual characteristics. There's no one universal remedy for flu, for example, because people differ from one another and so do their flus. You may have a flu with a severe sore throat, with inflammation and fever, and crave cold drinks. Your sister may have a flu with a sore throat that feels worse from swallowing and drinking anything at all. Each of you would require different homeopathic remedies to be treated most effectively.

POTENCY: LESS IS MORE

Homeopathic remedies are available in many different potencies, which are designated by a number followed either by the letter "c" (a centesimal scale) or an "x" (a decimal scale). Using the centesimal scale, one part of the original tincture is diluted with 99 parts of the base, which may be water or alcohol. Then one part of this dilution is further diluted with 99 parts of the base. This process continues until it produces solutions of 30c (30 dilutions) or 300c (300 dilutions), and so on. In the decimal scale, the one part of the original tincture is added to nine parts of the base, with 30x signifying 30 dilutions, for example. According to homeopathic theory, the higher the dilution, the greater the remedy's potency. For self-care, lower potencies in the range of 6c to 12c are usually recommended. Professional homeopaths usually prescribe higher potencies of 30c and more to treat deep-seated underlying conditions or severe emergencies.

How to Take Homeopathic Remedies

Follow the dosage directions on the product label; generally two to three pills or five to ten drops equals one dose. After taking a homeopathic remedy, you may notice some changes right away, or it may take time for symptoms to improve gradually.

Homeopathy comes with its own set of rules to follow. Although not all practitioners agree, most feel that to be safe and give homeopathy the best chance of working, it's best to follow these guidelines.

• Avoid touching the remedy with your hands, especially if you are giving it to another person. Rather, tip the required number of pellets into the container cap and then into the mouth; if tablets are blister-packed, pop them directly into the mouth. Touching the remedy could contaminate or inactivate it.

• The frequency of the dosage depends on the intensity of the symptoms: The more severe the symptoms, the more frequent the dose. You increase the potency by taking the same small dose more frequently; taking more pellets or drops per dose won't increase the potency.

• For severe symptoms, take the remedy every two to three hours for up to three doses; discontinue if you see improvement. Take another single dose if the symptoms recur. For mild symptoms, begin by taking one dose of the remedy only three times a day. As the symptoms improve or disappear, increase the interval between doses or stop the medication.

• Avoid eating or drinking anything for 15 to 30 minutes before and after taking the remedy. And allow it to dissolve slowly under your tongue so it is absorbed directly through your mucosa. (Some combination tablets instruct you to chew them instead.)

• Store homeopathic remedies in the original container, away from heat, sunlight, and strong-smelling substances that might contaminate them; the list includes perfumes, camphor and eucalyptus (found in many cosmetics and other items that inhabit a medicine chest, such as Tiger Balm, Vicks products, and lip balms), and mothballs. If you use a product containing eucalyptus or tea tree oil, use it several hours before or after each dose of a homeopathic remedy.

• Consult your health care practitioner before taking any homeopathic remedy, especially if you have any medical conditions or if you develop any adverse side effects.

If there is no improvement whatsoever after the first three doses, you probably have chosen the wrong remedy. Move down the list of recommended remedies, choose the next one that best fits your case, and repeat the dosing.

General Relief from Colds

A large number of homeopathic remedies are generally useful for colds; the following are the most commonly used. Allium cepa and Euphrasia are particularly suitable for summer colds, which tend to be milder than winter colds.

• *Aconite.* This remedy is sometimes called the vitamin C of homeopathy because it is most effective during the early stage of a cold, especially when the cold symptoms appear suddenly and violently after exposure to cold weather or wind; when there is a clear watery runny nose and a lot of sneezing; there may be a red, hot, dry sore throat, fever, and coughing; and the person may be restless and anxious but not delirious.

• *Allium cepa.* When the cold symptoms include a runny nose and eyes, which may be irritating and cause burning and redness (but not under the eyes); the larynx may tickle and there may be a dry, painful cough; symptoms are worse indoors, with warmth, and in the evening; better in the open air.

• *Euphrasia.* Helpful if the nasal discharge is clear, watery, and bland, while tears are irritating and there is redness under the eyes.

• *Mercurius.* For people with colds who are extremely sensitive to changes in temperature and easily become chilled or overheated. Their nights are restless and sweaty, but sweating does not make them feel better. They are intensely thirsty for cold drinks. They may have a painful sore throat, accompanied by fever, and the throat is red and swollen; the tonsils or throat may have white or yellow deposits of pus. They may experience a metallic taste in the mouth and drooling. Symptoms worsen with changes in temperature and when the person moves around; they are alleviated in moderate temperatures.

• *Nux vomica.* For colds with nasal congestion that is worse at night in a person who feels generally chilly and is irritable and impatient.

• *Pulsatilla.* Very useful for colds that have mainly nasal symptoms; mucus is thick, yellow or yellow-green, and nonirritating; it may smell bad and usually alternates with a thinner discharge; the nose may run in fresh air and in the morning, and become stuffy indoors and at night.

General Relief from Flu

Of the many remedies suitable for treating the flu, the following are most commonly used. Gelsemium is also useful for summer flus, which tend to be milder than winter flus.

• *Arsenicum.* For established flus in people who feel chilly and who sneeze violently and frequently; their noses feel ticklish and irritated and produce a watery discharge that irritates and burns the upper lip. Symptoms also may include fever, fatigue, and restlessness. There may be a dry hacking cough that burns with pain and which tends to spread to the chest. The person is thirsty for small sips of liquid and experiences restless sleep, especially around midnight. If a sore throat is present, it feels worse from swallowing, from cold beverages, and from cold air; it feels better from warm beverages. (Arsenicum may prevent chest involvement.)

• *Bryonia*. People who benefit from this remedy are irritable and achy and thirsty for cold liquids. They do not want to be moved or disturbed because of pain; they may have headaches that are worsened by almost anything: touch, movement, eating, talking, or just moving their eyes. Coughing often is a symptom; coughs are usually dry and racking, come on in fits and disturb sleep, and cause pain in the chest and abdomen; the cough is worse with any kind of movement, including breathing, eating, or drinking, although a sip of water may bring temporary relief. Symptoms are better with fresh or cool air or lying on the most painful side (usually the right side), and worse in warm rooms.

• *Gelsemium*. If the person is dizzy, droopy, drowsy and dull, think Gelsemium. This is the remedy for flu sufferers whose main symptoms are fatigue, extreme weakness, a heavy feeling in the limbs, and muscle pain; their eyeballs may ache and their eyelids feel heavy. There may be a low-grade fever, and they may feel chills along their back and feel chilly generally. Symptoms are worse with exertion because of weakness, and the person has little thirst.

• *Hepar sulphuricum*. For flus that appear after exposure to cold weather; the nasal discharge starts out as watery and then turns thick and yellow, smells bad, and drips down the throat; the throat feels as if there is a splinter in it and there may be spasms of coughing; the person feels chilly yet perspires and is sensitive to drafts, which trigger sneezing.

- *Mercurius.* (See page 151.)
- *Oscillococcinum.* Best used at the very first sign of flu to relieve symptoms of fever, chills, body aches, and pains.
- *Phosphorus.* For flu with profuse nasal discharge that may be one-sided, or when the nose is blocked, or when accompanied by a cough or fever. The cough is usually dry at night but may be loose and phlegmy during the day; there is usually chest pain or a feeling of a heavy weight on the chest; the larynx may feel raw, and the person may be awakened by the need to cough. Symptoms are worse with movement, changes in temperature, cold or fresh air, and lying down, particularly on the left side; symptoms are better with warmth.
- *Rhus toxicodendron.* For flu primarily characterized by extreme exhaustion and pains in the joints, bones, and legs; paradoxically, the person feels restless and worse if he or she lies still for long; accompanying symptoms include sleeplessness, nervousness, chilliness, thirst, sweating, and dry, hoarse throat. Symptoms are worse with initial movement but better with continued movement, such as a walk in the fresh air.

Relief for Specific Symptoms

Homeopathy also may be used to zero in on specific symptoms. Here are the most commonly used remedies for symptoms of fever, cough, sore throat, canker sores or cold sores, and sinusitis.

Fever

The following remedies are used most commonly to treat colds and flu when an intense, violent fever is the most prominent symptom.

• *Aconite.* When the fever has come on suddenly after the person became chilled; if symptoms include restlessness and anxiety and are worse at night; if the person feels hot on the inside but chilly on the outside; kicking the covers off is a common trait, as is unquenchable thirst.

• *Belladonna.* For the person who radiates heat and whose face is red and flushed; he or she may be excitable, spacey, and delirious. The person is thirstless yet may have a dry sore throat and a cough that may be very painful. The symptoms are worse in the afternoon, evening, and night.

• *Ferrum phosphoricum.* This is the remedy of choice when the symptoms are similar to those indicating Belladonna but are less intense.

Coughs

Many homeopathic remedies are used to treat coughs, each with its own symptom pattern. Several have already been described, including Aconite, Arsenicum, Allium cepa, Bryonia, Hepar Sulphuricum, Mercurius, and Phosphorus. The two following remedies also are commonly used but should be prescribed only if the cough is the predominant symptom and the person matches the pattern; otherwise stay with one of the general cold or flu remedies.

• *Antimonium tartaricum.* When there is rattling of mucus but little phlegm can be raised; great weakness and fatigue; especially useful in children.

• *Spongia*. This is often the remedy of choice for harsh coughs and the croup; the cough is dry, barking, and often compared with the sound of sawing through a dry log; the cough may wake the person at night; symptoms are worse during the day and with excitement, talking, or exercise; they are better with eating and drinking.

Sore Throat

If sore throat is the predominant symptom and is worse on one side, you may try one of the following most commonly used remedies.

• *Lachesis*. For painful, swollen throats that are worse on the left side or that spread from the left to the right. Symptoms are worse from drinking, particularly warm beverages, and worse in the morning or upon waking at night.

• *Lycopodium*. For sore throats that are worse on the right side; pain may spread from the right to the left; there is fever with chills. Throat pain is worse from cold air, but the person craves fresh air; the pain is better after a warm drink. Symptoms generally are worse in the late afternoon.

Note: Zinc lozenges that are specifically designed to dissolve easily may help hasten recovery and are compatible with homeopathy. However, avoid eucalyptus or mentholated lozenges if you are taking a homeopathic remedy, since these could serve as an antidote to the remedy.

Canker Sores or Cold Sores

Mouth sores of both types respond well to both oral and topical homeopathic medications, which may be used together.

ORAL REMEDIES

• *Mercurius.* For *canker sores* on gums, in the mouth, and on the tongue; when pain is stinging or throbbing; when the person secretes a lot of saliva; symptoms are worse at night. For herpes sores that itch, exude pus, form a crust, and are accompanied by swelling of the lymph nodes in the groin. The person is restless, hot, and chilly, and has a fever and night sweats.

• *Natrum muriaticum.* For *cold sores* that usually are found around the mouth and lips, the corners of the mouth, strung like little pearls. Natrum is also useful for *canker sores* that form on the gums.

• *Rhus toxicodendron.* For *cold sores* on the lips that burn and itch intensely, when symptoms include general malaise and achiness, and symptoms are better with warmth and worse with cold.

TOPICAL REMEDIES

• *Calendula.* For cold sores apply Calendula tincture diluted 10 drops in ½ cup sterile water, 3 to 4 times a day, to blisters that have opened, or use Calendula ointment. Canker sores may be soothed by using the same Calendula dilution as a mouthwash. DO NOT SWALLOW.

• *Urtica urens.* This remedy (stinging nettle) may be made as a tea and used as a wet dressing; or drink 2 to 3 cups of the tea daily if you are not taking another homeopathic remedy.

Sinusitis

The most often used homeopathic remedies for sinusitis are:

• *Kali bichromium.* When sinus pain occurs primarily at the root of the nose, in the forehead over one eye, and occasionally below the eyes. There is a very thick, puslike nasal discharge and crusts. Symptoms may begin in the morning, worsen by midday, and get better in the afternoon. The symptoms are worse from cold weather, bending down, and any motion such as walking; they are better from pressure, warmth, and drinking warm liquids.

• *Hepar sulphuricum.* For pain that occurs primarily at the root of the nose; the entire head may feel sore and bruised and sensitive to touch or movement; symptoms are worse from the cold air and in the morning. There may be a thick, offensive nasal discharge.

• *Silica.* For sinus pain that is worse from the cold, mental exertion, noise, motion, bending down, or talking; it is better with pressure and warmth. There is an irritating nasal mucus and crusts in the nose.

• *Mercurius.* (See page 151.)

Seeing a Professional Homeopath

In general, professional care is appropriate and preferable if self-care hasn't worked sufficiently or if you want to treat a serious condition. You also may feel safer and more confident practicing self-care if you have an established relationship with a homeopath whom you trust. That way, you have someone who knows you and with whom you can check to see if you are doing the right thing.

In homeopathy, there are essentially two types of disease or illness: acute (short-term) illness and chronic (long-term) illness. Colds and flu are acute diseases because the symptoms appear suddenly and are of relatively short duration. They are self-limiting, meaning that after they peak, they go away by themselves through the natural healing efforts of the vital force. Acute diseases are rather simple and easy to treat homeopathically.

COMBINATION REMEDIES

Should prescribing a single remedy prove too daunting (especially if you are miserable with symptoms and not thinking clearly), combination homeopathic remedies are an excellent alternative. They are more user-friendly because they are specifically labeled for colds and flu as well as specific symptoms such as sore throat or fever. Combination products contain two or more of the single remedies that are used most often to treat that symptom or condition. Therefore, this "shotgun" approach increases the chance that a product will contain the remedy you need, but at a low potency. Combination remedies are readily available at health food stores and pharmacies. As is the case with single remedies, if you don't get relief from a particular combination, don't give up on homeopathy. You may need to try another brand or two until you find the proper "fit." And if you still fail to see benefits, don't give up on homeopathy altogether—the combinations may not contain the particular remedy you require. You may need to consult a homeopathic physician for help in finding the right remedy.

Homeopathy is also useful in treating chronic, deep-seated conditions. If you suffer from frequent colds or flu, and the symptoms linger or turn into bronchitis or sinusitis, you may have a deep-seated immune problem. A professional homeopath will seek to treat the underlying disease with a *constitutional remedy*. Because chronic conditions are so entrenched, they usually take a long time to cure. Homeopathic remedies correctly prescribed for chronic disease strengthen your innate healing system and add to its knowledge. They gradually reduce the episodes of acute flare-ups while helping your mind-body to cure the underlying disturbance. As homeopathy cures, it also helps prevent future problems.

Healthy habits are important because the first rule in homeopathy is to "remove all obstacles to a cure." That's why most practitioners will act as health counselors and talk about the importance of nourishment on all three planes of existence. Homeopaths often advise on physical nourishment, which includes diet, exercise, rest, and vacation time; emotional nourishment, which includes relationships with other people and the free flow of feelings as the juice of life; and mental or spiritual nourishment, which includes learning, community involvement, and our relationship to the infinite of life and death.

As is the case with all medicine—conventional and alternative—most homeopathy in the United States is self-administered. However, according to the National Center for Homeopathy, there are about 3,000 homeopaths in this country. Of these, there are about 1,000 conventional medical doctors who practice homeopathy, 500 to 600 of whom practice it full time. Homeopathic physicians are licensed in only three states. Certification standards vary by profession—there is one certification for homeopathic M.D.'s and D.O.'s (doctors of osteopathy), another one for N.D.'s (doctors of naturopathy), another for D.C.'s (doctors of chiropractic). Your best bet is to find a health practitioner—medical doctor, nurse practitioner, or the like—who specializes in homeopathy and ask where they studied and how long they have been practicing homeopathy. It takes diligence, experience, and good intuition to succeed as a homeopath. There are two accredited colleges but no accredited medical schools in the United States devoted exclusively to homeopathy. Since homeopathic education takes place outside the conventional medical school system, homeopaths are likely to have irregular patterns of education. Generally, the more study time the better, and a homeopath usually should have a total of at least 500 hours of training, either through seminars, on-site and home-study training programs, or as part of the curriculum of a naturopathic college. The most sophisticated and comprehensive programs are given by the International Foundation for Homeopathy and the Hahnemann College of Homeopathy, which was formed by the Hahnemann Medical Clinic. (See Appendix A.) A homeopath should also continue his or her education after a formal training program has been completed, through seminars, workshops, home-study groups, and so on.

CHAPTER NINE

Mind-body Medicines

Why is it that a cold or flu usually arrives just when you can least afford to be sick? Or when you are feeling the most down? "Great, just what I need on top of everything else," you say with a groan. According to natural medicine, the timing should be no surprise, because stress and emotions play a central role in your immune system's response to viruses, bacteria, and many other forces associated with disease.

Throughout history, traditional folk medicines have acknowledged the connection between the body and the mind. Modern medicine took a brief vacation from this notion, diagnosing and treating body systems as separate entities and also considering the body to be independent of the mind. We now know that nothing could be further from the truth. Medicine is once again returning to the view that mind and body are one and together form something called the mind-body. This continual interplay between the physical and nonphysical aspects of your being is at the foundation of many of the natural healing arts.

In this chapter you'll see how science is learning to appreciate and manipulate the mind-body connection to improve immunity, even in advance of understanding exactly *how* these effects occur. And you'll learn how to reduce your susceptibility to colds, flu, and many other illnesses using relaxation techniques, stress management, laughter, meditation, guided imagery, and yoga. So stay upbeat, see a funny movie, seek out the small pleasures in life, help someone worse off than you are, and visualize your virus keeling over and dying. There's more to natural medicine than taking nutritional supplements, herbs, and homeopathic remedies . . . there's your mind.

Your Inner Healer

It's been said that no doctor ever cured anybody of anything. All a doctor does is set the stage and then step back to let the body heal itself. How this healing happens is anyone's guess. But there seems to be some vital inner force, or life force, that sparks and organizes our existence. It is suffused throughout our being and is the invisible thread that connects the physical, spiritual, and mental planes and keeps them healthy. Your inner force encompasses your innate power to heal and is central to many philosophies and forms of medicine; these include homeopathy, traditional Chinese medicine (where it is called *chi*), and Indian philosophy (where it is known as *prana* or *kundalini*). In the *Star Wars* movies, it was called simply "the Force."

Our innate power to heal ourselves has been underrecognized and underappreciated in conventional medicine; but you can see it in action when a placebo (sugar pill or fake medicine) is given. Often placebos are given to one group of subjects in an experiment, while another group gets the active or "real" medicine. The researchers then can compare the results of the two and see if the real medicine has any effect. Often the group taking the placebo shows improvement—30 or even 50 percent of the time—as well.

Physicians often dismiss this, trivializing it as "just the placebo effect," rather than giving this phenomenon its due respect. Instead of "placebo effect," we should be calling it "the self-healing effect." Many cases of "incurable" diseases have been cured without medical treatment, and many terminally ill people live way beyond their doctors' predictions. Such spontaneous remissions are examples of the healing efforts of this vital force at work.

Although there is much still to be learned, we do know that stress can have a tremendously detrimental effect on the healing force and be a factor in many ailments as big as cancer and as small as a cold. In fact, a pioneering study by Sheldon Cohen, a psychiatry professor at Carnegie-Mellon University in Pittsburgh, found that psychological stress could almost double the rate of respiratory infection—the higher the stress, the higher the risk.

Can Stress Cause Illness?

Dr. Hans Selye, the pioneering researcher who practically invented the concept of stress, defined it rather poetically: "Stress is anything from a passionate embrace to a boring game of chess." Stress can be a two-hour commute in bumper-to-bumper traffic, a marriage proposal, a job promotion, a *Die Hard*-type movie, a move to a new town, or news of yet another animal species becoming extinct.

We used to think psychological stress was all bad or

"negative." Now we understand that it is not the event itself, it is your *reaction* to the event that can be "negative." If you are unable to cope and feel overwhelmed instead of stimulated, threatened rather than challenged, helpless rather than in control—watch out: Stress could be opening the door to illness.

How stress does this is still being studied. We know that when we react to something in a negative way, an internal alarm goes off, triggering a cascade of physiological changes that Selye originally described as a fight-or-flight response. Adrenaline floods into the bloodstream, the heart beats faster, digestion screeches to a halt, muscles tense up, blood pressure skyrockets, the brain and senses become hyperalert. This response is designed to enable us to fight for our lives or to get us away from the danger as fast as possible. It worked well for our ancestors because their stressors were mainly of the saber-toothed tiger variety. Stresses were immediate and short-lived; once the dangerous situation was over, the body returned to normal.

Today life is not so simple or clear-cut. Instead of saber-toothed tigers, we're barraged by little day-to-day hassles—job insecurity or frustration, exasperating children, traffic jams, lack of fulfillment—that are difficult to fight or escape. When stress, even small stresses, becomes chronic, your adrenal glands steadily secrete cortisol to keep all systems on alert. Cortisol is difficult to metabolize. As a result of prolonged exposure to this stress hormone, your immune system is suppressed and your endocrine system gets worn down.

Nor is the stress response so simple and clear-cut. We now know that the way a person responds to stressful situations depends in part on the way he or she has learned to cope. Even the so-called negative emotions—

fear, anger, and so on—aren't necessarily harmful. Under certain conditions, these are all good, natural human emotions. But if they are not resolved, they become stressful. The more stress we perceive, and the less able we are to cope with it, the less we are able to recover from it, and the less we are able to deal with new stressors.

Prolonged stress wreaks all sorts of havoc: It can contribute to fatigue, diabetes, hypertension, ulcers, loss of libido, hormone imbalance, and reduced resistance to disease. Feeling stressed affects your ability to work, to think clearly, and to have satisfying social relationships. In 1993 the U.S. Public Health Survey estimated that 70 to 80 percent of Americans who visit physicians suffer from a stress-related disorder.

Psychoneuroimmunology

Today the notion that the thoughts in your mind have an enormous effect on your body has become so well accepted that there's even a tongue-twisting name for the new science that investigates the mind-body connection: psychoneuroimmunology, or PNI. Specifically, PNI studies the interaction among the mind, the nervous system, the immune system, and the endocrine system and acknowledges the unity of our complex interacting parts.

Early mind-body studies showed that people were more likely to become ill after suffering severe emotional trauma; recent studies have been able actually to measure the dip in immune defenses. In one study, the immune cells of students dropped significantly during exam week, presumably because of the extra stress. In another, rats were taught to shut down their own immune systems by conditioning alone. A study of seniors found that those who believed they were in poor health were about three times more likely to die within seven years than those who believed their health was excellent. In fact, what they *believed* their health to be was more accurate than their doctors' objective reports in terms of predicting death.

And perhaps most startling of all, a Stanford University Medical Center psychiatrist who set out to disprove the mind-body link provided strong evidence that it does exist. In the study, women with advanced breast cancer attended support groups in which they shared feelings and information and learned simple relaxation techniques. When compared with women who did not attend the groups, the supported women were less depressed, felt less pain, had a more positive outlook—and lived twice as long. Two of the women were still alive and disease-free ten years later, but none of the unsupported women survived. Many scientists suspect that the mind-body connection is involved in the documented spontaneous remissions from cancer and many other diseases that otherwise appear to be inexplicable.

As a result of these and other experiments, modern immunobiologists routinely refer to the immune system as a circulating nervous system. If stress exerts its effect by tiring out and depleting your nervous system and overworking the immune system, the key to stress and its ripple effect on the body is through the mind and nervous system. So the strategy is threefold: We can avoid and defuse stressful events, we can change the way we respond to them emotionally, and we can calm down an overchallenged nervous system with specific relaxation techniques.

Troubleshoot

The first thing you can do is evaluate your life stressors and change what you can. If your job is bringing you down, what can you do to fix it? Talk to your boss? Get more training and education so you can change jobs? What about your social relationships? Is something bothering you, or are you unsatisfied? Although maintaining the status quo may seem like the safest thing to do, consider that now might be the time to be brave, take the plunge, and bring troubles into the open.

Many people aren't even aware that a situation is stressful—we are conditioned to swallow anger and let hostility fester. Try this experiment. Take your "normal" pulse right now as you read this chapter. Then the next time you suspect you are feeling put upon, feel the side of your neck or your wrist for your pulse. Is it higher than normal? If so, your heart and immune system are being stressed, and it's time to get smart about defusing the situation.

Think Positive

How you perceive life in general influences your mood and, eventually, your health. A positive attitude seems to help your immune system resist a cold and shorten its duration, according to the work of Sheldon Cohen, the cold researcher who also found a connection between stress and colds. He found that the more positive people's attitudes, the less likely they were to catch colds and the milder the symptoms if they did come down with a bug.

Begin to change your attitude toward a more positive one. Pessimists expect bad things to happen and tend to dwell on them when they do. They perceive stress as something that is unpredictable and out of their control. Optimists expect good things to happen; they seek them out and remember them. They interpret "bad" events differently, thinking "This too shall pass, and it will probably set me free to find a job (or friend, spouse, or house) I like better.'' Try to find the lesson inherent in any situation, no matter how painful. Instead of the negative thought, look for a positive affirmative to help you avoid a recurrence.

It also may help to surround yourself with positive-thinking people. An intriguing experiment suggests that a positive attitude can be contagious—with enhanced immunity as a benevolent consequence. A professor at Harvard, David C. McClelland, studied students with early symptoms of a cold. Half were seen by an evangelistic healer who lavished them with personal, warm, sincere attention and told them they had the power to heal themselves. The other half were seen by the same healer but only briefly and impersonally and without the positive-thinking sermon. Amazingly, 11 out of the 13 in the first group had elevated IgA levels and shook off the cold. (IgA stands for immunoglobulin A, which is an immune system component that is a good indicator of resistance to respiratory illness.) But in the control group, the results were reversed: 11 out of 13 showed insignificant changes in IgA levels and did come down with colds.

Switch to Neutral

Variations in stress response occur because a stressful event is, in its broadest definition, any type of change or unexpected event. Your reaction to changes therefore may be positive, negative, or neutral. If you cannot switch to positive thinking, at least try to change the way you react to things so you no longer find them as stressful. Although no one likes to break a leg skiing, some people become greatly upset when this happens, while others remain a neutral calm and treat it as if it were the merest of ripples in their lives. People with "hardy" personalities are able to weather changes with equanimity and even zest. What some people would consider major tragedies they perceive as minor inconveniences or perhaps challenges to be met with energy and enthusiasm. While resistance to stress depends a good deal on your childhood experiences, you can develop more hardiness at any point in your life.

There are several ways to begin shifting from a tendency to react to stress negatively, to a more neutral or positive response. Try the following suggestions, adapted from the book *Healthy Pleasures,* by David Sobel and Robert Ornstein. With time, you'll evoke a healthier response, without suppressing your feelings and risking an explosive reaction later on. When something stressful happens to you:

- Avoid thinking in all-or-none terms. Be on the lookout for words like "all" or "completely": You are not totally stupid, and everyone else is not totally brilliant.
- Don't assume all situations are the same. They are not—and you always have the option of reacting differently.
- Don't assume the worst possible outcome. If you lose that client, it may not be as catastrophic as you imagine.
- Look for your strengths. In any situation, you probably show elements of both weakness and strength.
- Avoid blaming yourself for something that is beyond your control. Although we should accept personal responsibility when it's appropriate, blaming yourself for a party ruined by rain is not one of those times.
- Don't expect perfection in yourself and in others. Expecting perfection is a setup for failure and disap-

pointment. Everyone should do his or her best and strive to improve, but we learn more from our mistakes than from our successes.

- Imagine how any alternative reactions would make you feel and how you can use them to do better next time.
- Ask yourself: What difference will this make in a week, a year, or ten years? Some things just aren't that important when you take the long view.
- Consult your health care practitioner before taking an herb if you have any medical conditions or if you develop any adverse side effects.

Vive La Différence!

The story made headlines: A 1997 article in the *Journal of the American Medical Association* said that having a variety of different types of social relationships can help increase resistance to colds. Sheldon Cohen, who did the two studies on stress and positive attitude mentioned earlier, found that people with only one to three types of relationships had more than four times the risk of getting colds than those reporting six or more types of relationships. What's more, if they did get colds, those who knew many different types of people had the mildest symptoms—they produced less mucus, cleared nasal passages more effectively, and shed less virus than people with fewer types of social ties. The key was the *variety* of people—not the *number* of people—which points to a sense of community.

Many other studies show that people with multiple and diverse ties—friends, relatives, coworkers, neighbors—live longer than those with smaller social networks. So, the theory is that participation in a more diverse social network may temper a person's response to stress through promoting feelings of self-worth, responsibility, control, and meaning in life. Furthermore, we humans are social animals and need to feel connected with others, and feel warmly toward them.

Dr. Cohen found that a lack of diverse social contacts was a stronger risk factor than smoking, low vitamin C intake, and stress. That's why having close, intimate friends and significant others can be the most important step to take in preventing colds. Studies also suggest that isolation from other people and feelings of hostility damage the heart and that people who feel apart from their fellow humans are more likely to die of heart disease. When established relationships are disrupted owing, for example, to divorce or death of a loved one, people's health suffers. Even loving an animal is good for your health: People with pets report fewer minor health problems.

Laugh More, Sneeze Less

Ever since Norman Cousins used humor to help recover from a serious illness and wrote about it in his best-selling book, *Anatomy of an Illness,* researchers have been taking laughter more seriously. Lee Berk, a laughter researcher at Loma Linda University in California, has been studying the effects of laughter and believes that "mirthful" laughter is a kind of "eustress"—the opposite of "distress."

In contrast to distressful feelings such as anger and grief, which can suppress the immune system, eustress such as joy and laughter can strengthen it. In studies by Berk and others, laughter brought on by comedy video- and audiotapes elicited profound changes in the immune system—changes directly opposite those brought on by distress. Belly laughs increased levels of IgA antibodies, which protect the respiratory tract from the common cold.

Laughter also activated T-cells, which help fight infection; natural killer cells, which attack viruses, bacteria, and tumor cells; and gamma interferon, a chemical messenger that communicates among various immune components.

How does humor heal? Well, there are still plenty of gaps in our knowledge, but we do know that laughter engages the cerebral cortex—that part of the brain that contains pleasure centers and that may boost the immune system. Laughter also lowers stress hormones, which in turn affects the immune system. So, laugh more and you'll sneeze less. Put more humor in your life by socializing more (laughter is contagious, and people laugh more in the company of others); hang out with funny people; watch goofy cartoons instead of the nightly news. And the next time a cold or flu strikes, pop a video starring Steve Martin, Bette Midler, Jim Carrey, or other comedic clowns in the VCR. It may speed your recovery, but if not, at least it will make the time go faster.

The Faith and Caring Factor

If the ridiculous helps us resist colds, does the sublime? A growing body of evidence suggests that it does. Several studies demonstrate that having faith in a higher being and caring for someone other than yourself also can work immunological miracles. People who help others on a regular basis report fewer symptoms from colds, allergies, asthma, and autoimmune disease. Researchers in the field point to evidence that "helpers" experience a type of "rush" or "high" similar to the runners' high that is accompanied by a surge of endorphins. When their endorphin levels jump, they also experience a jump in immune power.

One researcher actually documented immune changes

that could influence the course of a cold. Steven Kelner discovered that study subjects who imagined themselves in a situation where they felt a "oneness with something larger than themselves" experienced an increase in IgA antibody levels.

This phenomenon is so powerful that, according to the work of David McClelland, just watching someone else be selfless is enough to switch on your immune system. Students who watched a film about Mother Teresa showed increased levels of IgA, whether they approved of her work or not!

Prayer also can play a role in your health—and that of others. In a review of over 200 studies on the effects of religious practice on health, more than half showed positive effects. For example, a cardiologist at San Francisco General Hospital designed a study in which one group of patients was prayed for and another group was not. Neither the patients nor their health practitioners knew which group was which. The patients who were prayed for did significantly better: They required less antibiotics, developed less pulmonary edema (fluid in the lungs), and were less likely to require insertion of a breathing tube. In several other experiments, subjects were able to stimulate or slow the growth of bacteria and fungi—from as far as 15 miles away! These and other intriguing experiments relating to prayer are documented in Larry Dossey's book, *Healing Words.*

Some scientists point out that people who pray are meditating, which in itself is a profoundly relaxing experience, and that this may account for some of the startling effects of prayer. But science has no way of explaining effects on people unknowingly being prayed for by others—or on bacteria!

The Pleasure Prescription: Lighten Up!

Take a good look at your life. Do you balance periods of challenging work with "down" times of rest and relaxation, of great and little pleasures? If not, you're not taking good care of yourself.

As Sobel and Ornstein write, "Doing 'nothing' and just hanging out is a vital part of self-renewal." In *Healthy Pleasures* they provide the scientific evidence for incorporating many other pleasures into our lives. Making love, eating delicious food, listening to pleasing music, and connecting with nature make us feel good and bestow relaxation and thus health and longevity. Advocates of common sense and moderation point out that people with stressful jobs need an outlet for their frustrations, not more frustration. Being forced to adhere to a strict diet, for example, actually worsened the health profile of hassled male executives, who saw this as one less thing they could control.

Paul Pearsall, in his book *The Pleasure Prescription,* advocates for "enlightened hedonism"—a life suffused with joy and a spiritual toughness that allows people to feel pleasure from every aspect of daily living. He points to work by Arthur Stone, at the State University of New York, who has documented the lasting immune-boosting power of simple, enjoyable activities such as having friends over for dinner, fishing, or even jogging. In a study in which 79 men chronicled their daily ups and downs, the appearance of cold symptoms coincided with a decrease in "desirable events" and an increase in "undesirable events" from three to five days beforehand—a period that covers the incubation period for the common cold.

Relaxation Techniques

We all can have the skills and make the time to relax as a normal part of our daily lives. Many, many ordinary activities and hobbies are relaxing—gardening, a walk in nature, exercise, adequate rest, and sleep. One approach to stress reduction—and immune health—includes specific relaxation techniques that calm the mind, and hence relax the body.

A study published in the journal *Psychosomatic Medicine* supports the notion that relaxation can boost immunity. Study subjects used either a relaxation technique similar to the Total Body Muscle Relaxation described on page 177, guided imagery (described on page 180), or simply lying down and turning their attention inward. After 20 minutes, the researchers found that all techniques boosted the level of IgA significantly, as compared with subjects who performed a simple task for 20 minutes. None worked better than the other, which suggests that it's important to find a technique with which you feel most comfortable.

Another study, performed at Harvard, compared a group that did deep breathing and progressive muscle relaxation and a group that did the same techniques but added guided imagery with a group that did neither. As expected, the group that did nothing showed no change in their immune systems. But those who practiced just the relaxation increased their levels of IgA. Those who did relaxation while imagining their T-cells attacking cold and flu viruses increased their IgA levels *and* their T-cells.

Are you so caught up in your responsibilities you just don't know *how* to let go? Help is at hand. The natural therapies that follow are designed particularly to help you easily and effectively reduce your stress reactions and give you increased peace of mind—and thus give a boost to your immune system. There's also evidence that these techniques can improve your ability to concentrate, relate to others, balance emotions, and open up to further personal growth.

Deep Abdominal Breathing

This simple technique helps reduce anxiety, depression, nervousness, muscle tension, and fatigue. It may be included as a part of total body muscle relaxation, meditation, and yoga. Loose-fitting comfortable clothes and dark, quiet surroundings help but are not required. You can try this anywhere, anytime you need to "take five."

1. To begin, sit or lie down in a comfortable position. Rest one hand over your abdomen and one on your upper chest. Take a few slow breaths and notice where your breath goes—does your chest rise and fall but not your abdomen? Or does your abdomen move alone? Which rises or falls first?

2. Next, breathe in slowly through your nose, attempting to fill your abdomen first, by lowering your diaphragm. This may take several tries for some people—imagine your torso is a balloon, expanding from the bottom first.

3. Once your abdomen is filled, keep inhaling and fill your chest, allowing it to expand in front, back, and sides.

4. Exhale slowly through your mouth, emptying first your chest and then your abdomen.

5. Repeat the inhalation and exhalation, trying to slow the breath even more. This should feel like a wave of air, rhythmically entering and leaving your body. En-

joy the turnaround times between the ins and outs of
your breath—this is your ''still point'' or ''gap'' of
higher consciousness and deeper relaxation.

Only breathing in should require any effort—allow the
air to flow out on its own as you let the weight of your
chest and abdomen relax down.

Total Body Muscle Relaxation

This is another basic technique that builds on the last
breathing exercise. Based on alternately tensing and relaxing your muscles, it effectively slows your breathing
and heart rate, leaving you rested and refreshed. Give
yourself 30 minutes to begin, and as you become adept,
you may reduce the time to 15 or 20 minutes. Begin in a
warm, quiet room; disconnect the telephone if possible.

1. Lying down, close your eyes and take a few deep
   breaths. Begin the deep breathing exercise described
   above and try to maintain it throughout the relaxation.
2. Focus your attention on your right foot and point
   your toes very hard. Hold for one slow breath and
   then let it go completely limp. Work up your right
   leg by flexing and relaxing your foot, tensing and
   relaxing your calf, and then tensing your thigh and
   then letting it go, enjoying the contrast between the
   two sensations. Then do your left foot and leg.
3. Now squeeze and relax your buttocks, waist, back,
   chest, right hand and arm, left hand and arm, shoul-
   ders, neck, and scalp. Include your face, opening
   your mouth and eyes wide, then scrunching them
   tight before completely relaxing those muscles.
4. Finally, stretch your arms and legs to their longest

length and elongate every muscle in between. Let go one more time.

5. Return your attention to your breathing and your surroundings, opening your eyes.

Meditation

Meditation has been integral to religions from Jewish mysticism to Roman Catholicism to Tibetan Buddhism. It is as varied as these religions and cultures are themselves, and has many goals, techniques, and effects. During meditation, the typical mental chatter ceases, at first for moments and then for minutes at a time with practice. During those moments, you experience the state of pure being, of oneness with the universe. Very interesting, you say—but what does this have to do with health?

In fact, hundreds of meditators have been studied and their physiological processes have been measured. At the very least, meditation has been shown to be deeply relaxing and rejuvenating. It lowers respiration, oxygen consumption, and metabolic rate. It reduces the blood levels of stress hormones, which are associated with immune suppression, poor health, and aging. Some long-term meditators have been found to be five to 12 years younger biologically than they are chronologically, as indicated by their blood pressure, visual acuity, and hearing.

There are many schools of meditation, but what they all have in common is the effort to focus the attention inward by concentrating on (meditating on) rhythmic breathing, an object, or a word, thought, or mantra such as the word "om." Or you focus outward on something such as a candle, a picture, God, or a space four feet in front of your nose. Meditation is a different experience for each person, and each session is different as well. The following exercise will help you get a glimpse of what meditation feels like. If you want to know more or explore this practice more deeply, there are many books and schools available.

1. Sit in a comfortable position that you can hold for as many as 10 to 15 minutes, in a quiet place where you won't be disturbed by the phone or other people.
2. Close your eyes; you may prepare yourself by doing the Deep Abdominal Breathing exercise described earlier. If you are very tense, do the Total Body Muscle Relaxation exercise.
3. Choose a word or phrase to focus your mind on, such as the ancient Sanskrit mantra *Ham Sah,* meaning "I am that"; or repeat the word "one" to yourself, or "I am love, I am joy, I am one." As you repeat the focus word(s) silently, thoughts will enter your head. When you catch yourself on a random thought chase, be grateful to your "observer self" for its observance and then let the seductiveness of your mental chatter recede. It is normal—no matter how many years of practice—for the mind to chase its own tail.
4. You can time your words or phrases with your breath, keeping the inhale broad, deep, and easy and the exhale silent and effortless.
5. You can easily lose track of time in deep relaxation, so you may need to set a timer or stopwatch if you don't have unlimited time.
6. Remain seated for a minute or two with your eyes closed, and then open them.

As simple as it sounds, some people find that sitting still and "doing nothing" is a very difficult assignment. So if you're the kind of person who usually buzzes around, doing 12 things at once, don't be surprised if you can't sit quietly or if your mind wanders. Keep with it, and don't be too harsh on yourself if you feel you aren't "doing it."

According to mind-body expert Joan Boryshenko, the meditation session itself is the goal; even if you think you're not doing it "right," the relaxation response is still likely to be occurring. She says that even beginners soon notice that they feel more peaceful. And the more they practice, the more adept they get and the better they feel. Aim to meditate once a day; twice if possible. The best time is when you wake up, when your mind is the most uncluttered and "suggestible." It's also nice to meditate again at the end of your workday, after exercising, and before a meal.

Guided Imagery

Guided imagery is a way of translating positive thoughts into mental images in order to achieve a specific result. It involves using your imagination—your "mind's eye"—to create internal visual images. Long used by competitive athletes to visualize their victory and give them a winning edge, this technique is now being used by medical patients to visualize health and wellness. For example, cancer patients mentally travel inside their bodies and picture the cells of their immune systems attacking cancer cells and the tumor gradually shrinking.

In recent research, subjects of Georgetown University psychologist Mary Banks Gregerson imagined their white blood cells attacking and ingesting weakened cold and flu viruses. When they focused on their blood, sure enough— blood lymphocytes went up. When they focused on their saliva, an immune component particular to saliva rose. Even children can learn guided visualization, as evidenced by a study in which children aged six to 12 were able to raise their IgA levels.

If you'd like to try visualization to marshal your immune system's antiviral forces, first put yourself in a state of deep relaxation using one of the techniques described earlier in this chapter. Then create your own unique image that embodies your immune system components patrolling your body and ferreting out viruses. Guided imagery is a very personal undertaking, and a particular image that works for one person does not always work for another. For example, for immune strengthening, you might try imagining your white blood cells as an army that attacks the viruses, and the viruses as weak and dying. Or you could concentrate on a particular symptom: If you have a fever, you could imagine yourself floating in a cool mountain lake.

Visualization is not easy for most people, at least at first. Some people never get the hang of it, but for others practice and persistence pays off. A professional imagery counselor certainly helps, and so can drawing on paper the images you are trying to imagine.

Yoga

Yoga derives from the Hindu religion and can be a spiritual practice that incorporates meditation and other mental exercises. There are many schools of yoga, but *hatha yoga,* which emphasizes physical postures called *asanas* and integrates them with breathing techniques, is the form most commonly practiced in Western countries, where it is available in health clubs, dance centers, and community centers.

Practicing hatha yoga regularly not only builds strength, flexibility, balance, and grace; it helps you reach a state of awareness, tranquility, and well-being. Yoga seeks to unite mind, spirit, and body. Regular practice helps balance and energize the entire body, including the immune, nervous, and endocrine systems. Recent evidence suggests it is just as good a stress reliever as vigorous aerobic exercise, and a lot gentler. Thus, it may help you reduce the frequency and severity of colds, flu, and other infections. Many studies have shown that yoga helps people reduce asthma attacks by relaxing the respiratory system.

Although it can be strenuous, yoga is highly adaptable to your abilities and is suitable for people of all ages. You can learn yoga from books and videotapes, but it's best to participate in yoga classes (or get individual instruction), especially if you're new to the practice. You may want to try the simple breathing exercise that follows. It is, first and foremost, supremely relaxing; as a side benefit, it also relaxes and strengthens the muscles you use to breathe.

ALTERNATE NOSTRIL BREATHING

For best results, use Deep Abdominal Breathing, described earlier, for the inhalations and exhalations.

1. Using your right hand, place your thumb next to your right nostril and your middle finger next to your left nostril. (See Figure 9.1.) Gently but firmly close off your right nostril with your thumb. Inhale through your left nostril, bringing your awareness to your heart.
2. Release your right nostril and close off your left nostril with your middle finger, exhaling through your right nostril.
3. Keeping your left nostril closed, inhale through your right nostril.

4. Close off your right nostril and inhale through your left nostril.
5. Repeat this breathing pattern 12 times.

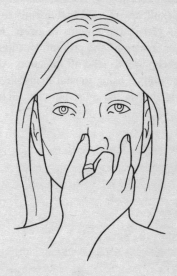

Figure 9.1

Physical Medicines to Reduce Stress

In addition to these mental approaches to stress reduction, there are many physical ways to interfere with the cycle of stress. Conventional medicine, for example, treats stress with antianxiety and tranquilizing drugs such as Valium—but these may be habit-forming and impose unwanted side effects. Instead, you may want to treat stress—both the initial psychological stress as well as the way your body responds physiologically—with natural remedies such as herbs (Chapter 7) and homeopathy (Chapter 8). For example, kava-kava, valerian, and linden flowers calm the nervous system; valerian, cramp bark, and chamomile relax tight muscles; and valerian, passion-flower, and skullcap are used traditionally to treat insomnia. Treating physical symptoms of stress may break the chain of stress reactions and prevent your immune system from losing its power to fend off infection. And taking the holistic approach of using mental medicine and physical medicine together is the most powerful antistress medicine of all.

CHAPTER TEN

Putting It All Together

Now that you know all about the possibilities and understand the rationale for using natural therapies to treat and prevent colds and flu, you may be thinking: "Whew! How do I put this all together into a practical program I can use?"

Obviously, you won't do *everything* covered in this book. But to do only one, such as just taking large doses of vitamin C or just taking the herb echinacea, would be a mistake. That's because no one approach is more effective than the others, and, as in conventional medicine, there are few (if any) single magic bullets that produce dramatic results when used all by their lonesome selves. Using a combination of approaches is more effective than any single effort and gives natural medicine a fair chance to work.

So, in the following programs, choose those elements that appeal to you the most and experiment with combinations to find out which is most effective for you. On the following pages, you'll find three step-by-step programs that outline exactly what to do. The first program is designed to be followed at the very first sign of a cold or flu to nip it in the bud. The second explains what to do if you have a full-blown cold or flu. The third is a prevention program to reduce the likelihood of your getting sick at all.

Treatment Program: At the First Sign

The best course of action is to stay ahead of the infection, when it is easier to treat. Learn to recognize the early-warning signs of an impending cold: dry, scratchy, tight throat; less-than-normal appetite; feeling slightly under the weather. They usually appear about 48 hours after the first viruses entered your respiratory system and up to 12 hours before the actual onset of symptoms. That way you can swing into action early, and you may be able to nip the cold in the bud. You'll have less warning with a flu, since symptoms generally come on more suddenly, two to three days after initial exposure. Still, the minute you feel that leaden, vaguely achy feeling, take action.

Many people who switch into "red alert" mode at the first sign and follow these steps find that they avoid getting sick at all or experience only mild symptoms for a few days. You, too, may be rid of your cold in two or three days instead of the typical seven; and your flu may be on its way in four to five days instead of ten to 14.

Begin on the morning of the very first day that you notice early warning signs. Don't forget to follow the basic home care strategies in Chapter 4, and continue this regimen until symptoms disappear, or unless otherwise specified. Even if you are not sure you have an infection coming on, or if you were just experiencing a bad night's sleep, you have nothing to lose by taking action, because these natural remedies are completely nontoxic in the recommended doses.

1. Take vitamin C supplements, up to 1,000 mg every one or two waking hours; reduce dosage if you experience bloating or diarrhea.
2. Take beta-carotene or mixed carotenoid supplements, 200,000 IU per day, in divided doses.
3. Take zinc gluconate lozenges, one every two hours, especially if you have a sore throat, for four to seven days.
4. Take an immune-stimulating herb such as echinacea, three times a day. You also may take an immune-stimulating mushroom extract or concentrate such as shiitake or maitake, plus the Chinese combination medicine Gan Mao Ling at the onset of a cold or Yin Ciao at the onset of a flu.
5. Take a homeopathic remedy. Aconite usually is recommended at the first sign of a cold and oscillococcinum at the first sign of a flu. (Note: Some homeopaths advise you not to use herbs, particularly strongly aromatic ones, if you use homeopathy.)

Treatment Program: So You Have a Cold or Flu . . .

Once an infection has settled in, it is more difficult to treat. Still, natural remedies can make a difference. If you get a full-blown infection, follow the basic home care strategies in Chapter 4, making sure you carefully follow precautions to avoid contagion. Then you also may take the following steps, until symptoms subside:

1. Take vitamin C supplements, up to 1,000 mg every one or two waking hours; reduce dosage if you experience bloating or diarrhea.
2. Take beta-carotene or mixed carotenoid supplements, 200,000 IU per day, in divided doses.
3. Take zinc gluconate lozenges, one every two hours, especially if you have a sore throat, for four to seven days.
4. Take an immune-stimulating herb such as echinacea, every two waking hours. You also may take an immune-stimulating mushroom extract or concentrate such as shiitake or maitake, and you also may wish to add the Chinese combination medicine Gan Mao Ling for a cold or Yin Ciao for a flu.
5. Take the appropriate homeopathic remedy; choose a single remedy as instructed in Chapter 8, or a commercial formula designed for colds or flu. (Note: Some homeopaths advise you not to use herbs, particularly strongly aromatic ones, if you use homeopathy.)
6. If you have strong symptoms, consider adding additional herbs for specific symptom relief. Try kitchen herbs such as basil for fever, black pepper for colds and sore throat, cayenne pepper for general relief, and fennel to expel mucus (Chapter 5). Or add medicinal herbs such as aniseed, balm of gilead, elecampane, and slippery elm for coughs; damiana or ephedra for congestion; boneset, lemon balm, or cayenne for fever (Chapter 7). If you are having trouble sleeping because symptoms are making you uncomfortable, take a natural sleep aid such as the herb valerian—sleep is one of the best healers. If you are prone to complications such as sinusitis or bronchitis, take goldenseal or astragalus three times a day.

Continue this regimen until you are well. Then gradually cut back the dosage of the herbs the following week until you are down to zero. Also gradually taper off the nutritional supplements until you are down to your baseline dose.

Postviral Care and Follow-up

If you've had the flu, avoid giving in to the temptation to jump right back into the swing of things the minute you feel better. The rule is: Wait one more day after you feel completely well before resuming anything resembling your normal level of activity. Ease into work, social activities, and exercise gradually, or you could give yourself a relapse. If you're recovering from a cold, you can begin resuming activities earlier, but try to take it easy the first day or two you're back at work.

If you do notice symptoms returning, immediately go back on the treatment program for a few days. Some natural medicine practitioners advise taking a postviral herbal tonic such as panax ginseng (page 138) to detoxify and build the immune system back up after an illness.

As you treat yourself or another person, be sure to write down the symptoms, each remedy you've used, as well as the results. Keep your notes as part of the family's home health file. An ongoing health file provides you with a valuable record and better enables you to prescribe effective remedies next time. If that person gets a cold or flu again next year, you can check through the file to see what worked and what didn't. Each family member may respond differently to the various forms of therapy, with one responding beautifully to general home care, homeopathy, and nutritional supplements; another responding best to echinacea, aromatherapy, and guided imagery.

Prevention Program

The best course of action is to pay attention to your physical and mental health all year round. Failing that, beginning at least one month before and continuing through the cold and flu season, follow this basic plan.

1. Follow the "Eight Strategies to Boost Immunity" in Chapter 3.
2. Upgrade your diet to include foods rich in vitamins, minerals, and omega-3 essential fatty acids—mostly fresh fruits and vegetables, whole grains, nuts, flax-seed oil, and beans—and low in fat, refined sugars, and artificial food additives. Try to find locally grown organic food, if possible.
3. Take a multivitamin-mineral supplement every day that supplies at least the RDAs, and preferably higher. You may add extra vitamin C, beta-carotene (or mixed carotenes), vitamin E, selenium, and flavonoids, plus garlic and omega-3 fatty acids.

If you have gotten several colds or flu in the past, you may have a compromised immune system, so you may want to add the following for extra insurance:

1. Take a tonic herb to boost immunity, such as echinacea, astragalus, or ginseng throughout the flu season (November through January). If a single herb does not improve immunity enough to prevent colds and flu, try using the tonic combination (page 138) or adding one or more of the medicinal mushrooms described in Chapter 5.
2. If you get a lot of mucus and lung congestion or bronchitis, or have lung disease, you may take 1,000

to 1,200 mg of the amino acid N-acetylcysteine, in divided doses, as a preventive.

3. If you still find you are getting colds and flu every year, consider working with a naturopathic physician, nutritionist, herbalist, homeopath, or traditional Chinese medicine practitioner to treat what may be a deep-seated weakness in your immune system.

Resources

To learn more about natural therapies or to obtain referrals to practitioners near you, contact the following organizations. To obtain products through the mail, contact the following reputable mail-order sources.

General Information

Alliance for the Prudent Use of Antibiotics
P.O. Box 1372
Boston, MA 02117
617-636-0966

American Association of Naturopathic Physicians
2366 Eastlake Avenue, East Suite 322
Seattle, WA 98102
206-323-7610
Send $5 for a brochure and list of doctors.

American Association of Oriental Medicine
433 Front Street
Catasauqua, PA 18032
610-266-1433
Call or write for a list of acupuncturists who meet their standards.

American Holistic Medical Association
6728 Old McClane Drive
McClane, VA 22107
703-556-9728; 703-556-9245
Send $10 for a member directory.

Centers for Disease Control and Prevention
Center for Infectious Diseases
Div of Viral Diseases
1600 Clifton Road, NE
Atlanta, GA
404-639-3574

Herb Organizations

The American Botanical Council
P.O. Box 201660
Austin, TX 78720
800-373-7105 for catalog
512-331-8868
http://www.herbalgram.org

The American Herbalists Guild
P.O. Box 746555
Arvada, CO 80006
303-423-8800

Herb Research Foundation
1007 Pearl Street, Suite 200
Boulder, CO 80302
303-449-2265
800-307-6267 orders only
http://www.herbs.org

Herbal Products

Herbal products are available at health food stores, pharmacies, and herb stores. The following have a reputation for high-quality products; write or phone for information about your nearest distributor or about ordering herbs by mail.

East-West Herb Products
65 Mechanic Street, Suite 103
Red Bank, NJ 07701

East Earth Trade Winds
P.O. Box 493151
Redding, CA 96049
800-258-6878 for catalog
916-223-2346
http://www.snowcrest.net/eetw/
Chinese herbal formulas

Eclectic Institute, Inc.
Sandy, OR
503-668-4120; 800-332-4372
www.eclecticherb.com
Organic herbs

Herb-Pharm
P.O. Box 116
Williams, OR 97544

Herbs for Kids
Bozeman, Montana
406-587-0180
Certified organic and pesticide- and alcohol-free herbs
formulated for children

Nature's Herb Company
Box 118, Dept. 34,Q
Norway, IA 52318
800-237-0869

Planetary Formulas
P.O. Box 533W
Soquel, CA 95073
800-606-6226

Rainbow Light
207 McPherson Street, Dept. P
Santa Cruz, CA 95060
888-669-7766

TransPacific Health Products
3924 Central Avenue
St. Petersburg, FL 33711
800-336-9636
Chinese herbal formulas

Homeopathy Organizations

American Institute of Homeopathy (AIH)
801 N. Fairfax St., Suite #306
Alexandria, VA 22314
703-273-5250

John Bastyr College of Naturopathic Medicine
14500 Juanita Drive NE
Bothell, WA 98011
206-823-1300

Hahnemann Medical Clinic
828 San Pablo Avenue
Albany, CA 94706
510-524-3117

International Foundation for Homeopathy (IFH)
P.O. Box 7
Edmonds, WA 98020
425-776-4147

National Center for Homeopathy (NCH)
801 N. Fairfax Street, Suite 306
Alexandria, VA 22314
703-548-7790

National College of Naturopathic Medicine
049 SW Porter St.
Portland, OR 97201
503-499-4343

Homeopathic Remedies

Homeopathic remedies are available in a growing number of health food stores and pharmacies. If you cannot locate a local supplier for the remedies you need, the following companies will send individual remedies to you by mail; many also supply homeopathic remedy kits and books on homeopathy.

Boericke and Tafel, Inc.
2381 Circadian Way
Santa Rosa, CA 95407
800-876-9505

Boiron, USA
800-BLU-TUBE
800-264-7661 Consumer
Information Line

Dolisos America, Inc.
3014 Rigel Avenue
Las Vegas, NV 89102
800-365-4767

Hahnemann Medical Clinic
828 San Pablo Avenue
Albany, CA 94706
510-524-3117

Homeopathic Educational Services
2124 Kittredge Street N
Berkeley, CA 94704
800-359-9051
510-649-0294

Humor Therapy

The American Association of Therapeutic Humor
222 South Merrimac, #303
St. Louis, MO 63105

Mind-Body Healing

Center for Mind-Body Medicine
5225 Connecticut Avenue, NW, Suite 414
Washington, DC 20015
202-966-7338

Institute for the Study of Human Knowledge
P.O. Box 176
Los Altos, CA 94023
   Publishes a newsletter, *Mental Medicine Update,* edited
by David Sobel, M.D. and Robert Ornstein, Ph.D.

Yoga

Yoga Journal
2054 University Avenue
Berkeley, CA 94704
   A comprehensive yoga resource, with articles and list-
ings of classes and workshops nationally.

Glossary

Acupuncture—A technique used in traditional Chinese medicine that punctures the skin with thin needles at certain points of the body in order to manipulate the *chi,* or life force. In acupressure, no needles are used; rather, fingers are used to press the points.

Adrenaline—A hormone released by the adrenal glands during times of stress.

Allopathic medicine—A system of medicine that uses treatments that have the opposite effect from that which is caused by the disease or injury. Often it entails suppressing the symptoms rather than treating the underlying condition. Also called conventional or mainstream medicine.

Antibody—A protein molecule made by B-cells that identifies a particular foreign body such as a virus, inactivates it, and marks it for destruction by other white cells of the immune system.

Antigen—A substance that identifies a substance that is foreign to the body (nonself), which causes the body to form an antibody that responds to it specifically.

Antihistamine—A substance that reduces the effects of histamine, a chemical made by the body in response to a foreign substance (allergen).

Antioxidant—A molecule made by the body or eaten as a food or supplement that chemically prevents oxidation of cells by free radicals.

B-cells—White cells of the immune system that are produced in the bone marrow and that produce antibodies.

Botanicals—Medicines derived from plants, including herbs.

Bronchitis—Inflammation of the mucous membranes of the lungs.

Cilia—Tiny hairs that line the respiratory tract and sweep viruses and other particles caught in mucus down to the stomach for destruction.

Cold—A contagious viral infection of the upper respiratory tract, usually minor in nature.

Complement—Protein molecules released when an antibody locks onto an antigen and that penetrate the outer shell of the foreign body.

Decoction—A strong brew of herb tea made by boiling and then steeping the root and bark in water.

Extract—A concentrated herbal preparation made with water.

Flavonoids (bioflavonoids)—A group of chemicals found in plants that are helpful in many essential body functions, including protection from free radicals.

Free radical—An unstable molecule lacking an electron that steals an electron from other molecules in cells of the body, thus harming the cells, including those of the immune system.

Guided imagery—A form of self-therapy in which a person creates an image in his or her mind of a desired outcome, such as white cells destroying a virus.

Helper T-cells—White blood cells that patrol the bloodstream, recognizing antigens and alerting other components of the immune system.

Histamine—A compound that cells release as part of the immune response to a harmful foreign body, such as a virus. This allergic reaction causes inflammation, increased blood flow, and mucus production.

Homeopathy—A system of medicine based on the principle of "like cures like"; it treats a person by administering a very small dose of a medication that would bring on the symptoms of the disease if taken by a healthy person.

Immune system—A complex system that protects the body from infection and other diseases. It is composed of the various types of white blood cells and the lymphatic system, which includes the thymus gland, lymph tissues, and spleen.

Immunoglobulins—Five distinct antibodies formed in response to certain antigens; immunoglobulin A (IgA) is the most common and is the major immunoglobulin found in the mucosa, where it defends the body against invading microorganisms such as viruses.

Influenza (or flu)—A highly contagious viral infection of the upper respiratory tract that may be serious.

Infusion—The most common method of preparing herb tea, made by pouring boiling water over the petals, flowers, or leaves and allowing it to steep.

Interferon—A protein released by cells that are under attack by viruses; it protects neighboring cells from infection.

Interleukin 1—A protein of the immune system that activates T-cells and macrophages and causes inflammation and fever.

Leukocytes—White blood cells.

Lymphocytes—T-cells and B-cells that arise from the lymph glands; they are usually about 25 percent of the total white cell count but increase in number when there is an infection.

Macrophages—Large white blood cells that patrol the body, surrounding and digesting foreign substances, such as viruses.

Mucosa—Mucous membranes that line the inside surface of air passages, containing mucus glands that secrete mucus.

Natural killer cells—T-cells that attack and destroy viruses and other nonself particles, including cancer cells.

Naturopathic medicine—A form of natural healing that treats the whole person, including the mind, body, and spirit.

Phagocytes—White blood cells that scavenge and mop up debris after other immune system components have done their job.

Phytochemicals or phytonutrients—A group of chemicals contained in plant foods (fruits, vegetables, herbs) that have a beneficial effect on health; phytochemicals and their functions are still being discovered.

Placebo—An inactive substance given as if it were a real dose of a drug; often used in drug studies to compare the effects of the inactive substance with those of an experimental drug.

Prostaglandins—Hormonelike fatty acids that have a variety of functions, including inflammation.

Rhinovirus—The type of virus that causes most colds; there are over 200 varieties.

Sinusitis—Inflammation of the mucous membranes of the sinuses, caused by either a viral or a bacterial infection.

Suppressor T-cells—White blood cells that wind down the immune response after it has dealt with an infection.

T-cells—White blood cells made in the bone marrow that mature in the thymus gland.

Tincture—A concentrated herbal preparation made with alcohol.

Virus—A tiny bundle of genetic material surrounded by a protein capsule, which is capable of invading a living cell and using it to replicate thousands of copies of itself.

For Further Reading

Bauer, Cathryn. *Acupressure for Everybody*. New York: Henry Holt, 1991.

Brown, Donald. *Herbal Prescriptions for Better Health*. Rocklin, CA: Prima Publishing, 1996.

Bruning, Nancy. *The Natural Health Guide to Antioxidants*. New York: Bantam, 1994.

Bruning, Nancy and Weinstein, Corey, M.D. *Healing Homeopathic Remedies*. New York: Dell Publishing, 1996.

Castleman, Michael. *The Healing Herbs*. Emmaus, PA: Rodale Press, 1991.

Castleman, Michael. *Nature's Cures*. Emmaus, PA: Rodale Press, 1996.

Castro, Miranda. *The Complete Homeopathy Handbook*. New York: St. Martin's Press, 1990.

Colbin, Annemarie. *Food and Healing* New York: Ballantine, 1986.

Cummings, Stephen, and Ullman, Dana. *Everybody's Guide to Homeopathic Medicines: Taking Care of Yourself and Your Family with Safe and Effective Remedies*. Los Angeles: J.P. Tarcher, 1991.

Elias, Jason. *The A-to-Z Guide to Healing Herbal Remedies.* New York: Dell Publishing, 1995.

Fezler, William. *Total Visualization: Using All Five Senses.* Englewood Cliffs, NJ: Prentice-Hall, 1992.

Ford, Norman D. *Eighteen Natural Ways to Beat the Common Cold.* New Canaan, CT: Keats Publishing, 1987.

Gach, Michael Reed. *Acupressure's Potent Points.* New York: Bantam Books, 1990.

Hendler, Sheldon Saul. *The Doctor's Vitamin and Mineral Encyclopedia.* New York: Fireside/Simon & Schuster, 1990.

Ivker, Robert. *Sinus Survival,* 3rd ed. Los Angeles: JP. Tarcher, 1995.

Krieger, Delores. *Accepting Your Power to Heal: the Personal Practice of Therapeutic Touch.* Santa Fe, NM: Bear, 1993.

Lappe, Marc. *When Antibiotics Fail: Restoring the Ecology of the Body.* Berkeley, CA: North Atlantic Books, 1995.

Lieberman, Shari, and Nancy Bruning. *The Real Vitamin & Mineral Book,* 2nd ed. Garden City Park, NY: Avery Publishing Group, 1997.

Mindell, Earl. *Earl Mindell's Herb Bible.* New York: Simon & Schuster, 1992.

Murray, Michael. *The Healing Power of Herbs,* 2nd ed. Rocklin, CA: Prima Publishing, 1995.

Namikoshi, Toru. *The Complete Book of Shiatsu Therapy.* New York: Japan Publications, 1981.

Pearsall, Paul. *The Pleasure Prescription: To Love, to Work, to Play—Life in the Balance.* Alameda, CA: Hunter House, 1996.

Tierra, Michael. *The Way of Herbs.* New York: Pocket Books, 1990.

Weil, Andrew. *Natural Health, Natural Healing.* Boston: Houghton-Mifflin, 1990.

References

McCaleb, Rob. "Straight Talk on Herbs." *Natural Health* (March-April 1997): 42–46.

"Psychological Stress and Susceptibility to the Common Cold."
New England Journal of Medicine 325 (1991): 606–612.

"Should Children Always Be Given Antibiotics for Acute Ear
Infection?" *Health Facts* (newsletter of the Center for
Medical Consumers) 22, no. 7 (July 1997): 3–4.

"Social Ties and Susceptibility to the Common Cold." *Journal
of the American Medical Association* 277, no. 24, (June 26,
1997): 1940–1944.

"Zinc Gluconate Lozenges for Treating the Common Cold. A
Randomized, Double-Blind, Placebo-Controlled Study."
Annals of Internal Medicine 15 (July 1996): 81–88.

Index

ABOUT THE AUTHOR

Nancy Bruning is a freelance writer specializing in health, nutrition, fitness, and the environment. She is the author or coauthor of many other books, including *Coping with Chemotherapy* (Ballantine Books, 1992); *The Natural Health Guide to Antioxidants* (Bantam, 1994); *The Real Vitamin & Mineral Book* with Shari Lieberman, Ph.D. (Avery Publishing, 1995); *Breast Implants: Everything You Need to Know* (Hunter House, 1995); *Healing Homeopathic Remedies* (Dell, 1996); and *The Mend Clinic Guide to Natural Medicine for Menopause and Beyond* (Dell, 1997). Bruning also writes articles for national magazines and patient education brochures. She is a native New Yorker who currently lives in San Francisco.